MAGDALENE
MANIFESTATION CARDS

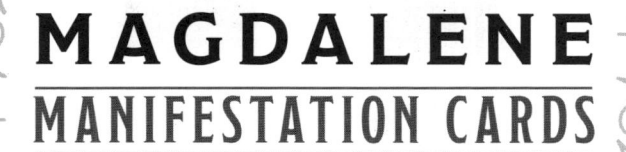

Create Abundance through Love

DANIELLE RAMA HOFFMAN

Artwork by Christine Lucas

Bear & Company
Rochester, Vermont

Bear & Company
One Park Street
Rochester, Vermont 05767
www.BearandCompanyBooks.com

Bear & Company is a division of Inner Traditions International

Copyright © 2023 by Danielle Lynn Hoffman

All rights reserved. No part of this book may be reproduced or utilized in any form or by any means, electronic or mechanical, including photocopying, recording, or by any information storage and retrieval system, without permission in writing from the publisher.

ISBN 978-1-59143-480-1 (print)

Printed and bound in China by Reliance Printing Co., Ltd.

10 9 8 7 6 5 4 3 2 1

Text design by Virginia Scott Bowman and layout by Kenleigh Manseau
This book was typeset in Garamond Premier Pro with Majesty and Modesto used as display typefaces
Artwork by Christine Lucas

To send correspondence to the author of this book, mail a first-class letter to the author c/o Inner Traditions • Bear & Company, One Park Street, Rochester, VT 05767, and we will forward the communication, or contact the author directly at **https://daniellehoffman.com**.

The Magdalenes and I dedicate this card deck and guidebook to you. We infuse them with divine love and calibrate them with the higher purpose of opening the heart and the return of divine wholeness. We welcome you into this sacred temple that is the Magdalene Codes of Love living transmission from a place of equality and as an adept, a Magdalene, an ambassador for love. We call upon the elements of Air, Water, Fire, Earth, and Akasha and the 100 percent pure love and light beings that are pertinent to you and your walk on this Earth to assist you in creating abundance through love. May you walk in beauty and your mission be buoyed by physical resources of overflowing love, money, energy, and relationships.

It is so and so it is!

Contents

Acknowledgments   xi

Preface: The Origin of This Body of Work   xiii

A NEW PARADIGM OF MANIFESTING

Meet the Magdalenes   2

Five Spiritual Truths of 5D Manifesting
  as a Magdalene   8

How to Use This Manifestation Deck:
  A Multidimensional Love Technology   19

CARD DESCRIPTIONS

Four Resource Codes

1 Yummy Money   34
  • *Resource—Thriving Mission*   35

2 Sublime Time   38
  • *Resource—Highest Timeline*   40

3 Divine Relationships   43
  • *Resource—Vibrational Leadership*   45

4 Radiant Energy — 48
- *Resource—Opulent Vitality 50*

Twenty Codes of Love

5 Love Conception — 54
- *Key—Ensouled Creations 56*
- *Hologram—Optimal Environments 57*

6 Magdalene Molecule — 60
- *Key—Confident Creator 61*
- *Hologram—Power of Community 62*

7 Birthright of Love — 66
- *Key—Authentic Expression 67*
- *Hologram—Openhearted Connection 69*

8 Ecstatic Bliss — 73
- *Key—Joyful Simplicity 74*
- *Hologram—Signature Essence 76*

9 Temple of Love — 78
- *Key—Physical Radiance 79*
- *Hologram—Vibrant Home 81*

10 Infinite Love Meridian — 84
- *Key—Structured Flow 85*
- *Hologram—Infinite Supply 87*

11 Star Love — 90
- *Key—Stellar Gifts 91*
- *Hologram—Deep Belonging 93*

12 Magic of Love — 96
- *Key—Miraculous Results 97*
- *Hologram—Crystal Clarity 98*

13 Magdalene Heart — 101
- *Key—Magnificent Receiver 102*
- *Hologram—Circulate Abundance 103*

14 Emerald Love — 106
- *Key—Stabilized Expansion 107*
- *Hologram—Bespoke Nourishment 108*

15 Orgasmic Creation — 111
- *Key—Blissfully Fulfilled 113*
- *Hologram—Ecstatic Wealth 114*

16 Magdalene Love Body — 117
- *Key—Multi-D Communication 118*
- *Hologram—Vibrational Autonomy 120*

17 Embodied Radiance — 122
- *Key—Divinely Glowing 123*
- *Hologram—Physically Energized 124*

18 Heart-Sentience — 128
- *Key—Higher Knowing 129*
- *Hologram—Mega Manifester 131*

19 Multi-D Abundance — 134
- *Key—Aligned Growth 135*
- *Hologram—Simultaneous Wealth 138*

20 Exponential Expansion — 140
- *Key—Energetic Preparation 141*
- *Hologram—Quantum Leap 143*

21 Source Union — 146
- *Key—Re-Sourced Wealth 147*
- *Hologram—Divine Connection 149*

22 Vibrational Visibility — 152
- *Key—Highly Magnetic 153*
- *Hologram—Empowered Potency 154*

23 Fully Realized — 157
- *Key—Manifestation Master 158*
- *Hologram—Spiritual Adeptness 160*

24 Magdalene Love Being — 162
- *Key—Akashic Manifesting 163*
- *Hologram—Love Ambassador 164*

CARD SPREADS AND MANIFESTATION VORTEXES

How to Use the Card Spreads — 168

- *One-Card Spread—Daily Support 171*
- *Two-Card Spread—Feminine-Masculine Alignment 172*
- *Three-Card Spread—Manifest While You Sleep 174*
- *Five-Card Spread—Long-Term Projects 176*
- *Wild Card Spread—Divinely Guided 178*

Resource Codes Spreads — 179

- *Sixteen-Card Spread—Create Multi-D Abundance 180*
- *Yummy Money Spreads— Actualize a New Paradigm of Wealth and Create an Extraordinary Partnership with Yummy Money 181*
- *Sublime Time Spreads— Unlock Your Sublime Time Treasure Chest 185*
- *Divine Relationships Spreads— Call In or Upgrade Relationships 187*
- *Radiant Energy Spreads— Regenerate, Rejuvenate, and Renew 190*

Conclusion: Deepening Your Magdalene Manifestation Practice — 194

※

What's Next: Explore Additional Ways to Work with the Magdalenes — 196

About the Author and the Artist — 201

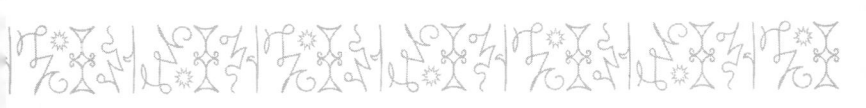

Acknowledgments

I love the art of appreciation. It cultivates a yummy feeling, activates a high vibe, and is a core part of my successful manifestation practice. As you read I invite you to receive the energy of appreciation imbued into these words. Thank you for choosing to enter into this sacred text and your contribution to the evolution in consciousness.

A special shout out to my Divine family—our clients at Divine Transmissions—past, present, and future. It is a blessing and an honor to walk this path with you. Much love to you from my heart to yours.

A heart-felt wave of gratitude to all the lightworkers, coaches, and mentors that have been a part of my rapid growth, for all the good you do in the world. To the extraordinary Elizabeth Purvis, thank you for helping me ground and translate the galactic vibey language of the guides onto Earth to reach even more souls. To Josiane Froment and my French spiritual sisters, thanks for modeling unconditional love.

Birthing the Magdalene Manifestation Cards was a team effort and a joy to cocreate with purpose-driven souls. Oodles of appreciation to artist Christine Lucas for our aligned partnership and for these gorgeous cards. To my operations manager Tara Dunion, thank you for our more than a decade strong partnership and for assisting me in making an even bigger difference on the planet. Thank you branding alchemist Carol Hampshire for the elegant website design and our brand colors, which inspired the beautiful book cover.

To the entire publishing team at Inner Traditions, praise for your expertise in all things books and deep appreciation for the ripple effect that having these published works in the world has in reuniting aligned souls across the globe. Special thanks to all of you who worked on this project, including Jon Graham, Erica B. Robinson, Patricia Rydle, Manzanita Carpenter, Renée Heitman.

Infinite love to my friends, family (two-legged and four-legged), and the guides for your love. Thank you beloved Friedemann for sharing your life with me. You have one of the biggest hearts I have ever seen and I am illuminated in the glow of your love. I love you! Thank you to the Magdalenes for hand-delivering this incredible manifestation curriculum for lightworkers around the globe to thrive and fulfill the missions we incarnated for. It takes all of us (beings in light and in form) to raise consciousness together.

Preface
The Origin of This Body of Work

A Note from Danielle
Scribed on 12/21/21 in Southern France

Dear priestesses and priests of Isis, Nephthys, and the Magdalene lineages: In 2002 I was called home to Egypt for the first time (in this body). One night, after a splendid evening watching bliss-faced Sufi dancers spiraling their devotion to the Divine, I saw Thoth, a being of light, with my eyes wide open. I have to admit that part of me was kind of freaked out while the rest of me was in awe of this incredibly mystical experience.

This wasn't my first encounter with Thoth, for we initially met in this lifetime in 1996. We had been deeply connected on the energy planes for about three years prior to my being in Egypt and I recognized his signature energy. However, this was the one and only time that, rather than seeing him in my mind's eye, I saw him with my physical eyes. I knew this was a special moment in our partnership. Our exchange only lasted a few minutes, however, I sensed that I was receiving many tablets of higher wisdom; bodies of work that we were to unpack together.

My love for Egypt, although not something I was interested in before my early thirties, became all-consuming. My beloved husband, Friedemann, and I began leading tours there, and went back a dozen times between 2002 and 2011. Each time that we visited the temple of Philae, dedicated to the goddess Isis, for a private visit before sunrise, my heart swelled with excitement and a sense of wonder and gratitude. I adored being the first to walk into the temple in the darkness, for I have always loved the nighttime. Each step took me closer and closer to the holy of holies and into the wings of Isis and her sister Nephthys (who is associated with the nighttime).

Each ceremony was potent, loving, and magical. After the group left the temple to watch the sunrise, I would stay in the holy of holies, sitting on the floor behind the altar stone.

Sometimes I cried the grief of a thousand lifetimes, while at other times I meditated so deeply I wasn't sure if I was sleeping. I talked openly with Isis and Thoth about my mission and purpose. Every time my mom or Friedemann came to get me to leave, I felt like I was being pulled from the womb. I was thirsty for more—more love, more magic, more space in which to steep. Each time we left Egypt this sensation of not being ready to leave compounded. I had an unquenchable thirst and divine calling to go deeper into Source.

This Egyptian decade was incredible, during which I received a few requests from Thoth and the Divine—what I like to think of as divine assignments. The first was to scribe *The Temples of Light: An Initiatory Journey into the Heart Teachings of the Egyptian Mystery Schools.* This was followed by *The Council of Light: Divine Transmissions for Manifesting the Deepest Desires of the Soul*. Both were requests to cocreate, to which I joyously said yes.

I became more curious about creation—creating bodies of work with Source and creating in the physical realm. I embarked on a passionate exploration of the art of manifesting. How do we create? What was the process of bringing an idea into form? What role does our connection to energy, Source, and our guides play? How can we consistently manifest our deepest desires?

Fast-forward to our 2011 Egypt tour. Surprisingly, when we left Egypt this time, I felt ready to go home. I had a deep sensation of completing an essential initiatory cycle into a level of adeptness. The deepest calling of my soul was taking me in a new, unexpected direction—to southern France. In 2012 we packed up our two kitties and moved to France. I was keenly aware of the connection between Egypt and France. Isis and her priestesses and priests had journeyed from Egypt to France; these adepts had included the Magdalenes (Mary Magdalene, Yeshua) and many others.

Although I was aware of Mary Magdalene at that time, I didn't have a strong connection with her. Our dynamic was more like a sisterhood, a recognition of the initiations we'd participated in with Isis in Egypt. My access to the love lineages had originated with Isis, and chronologically this felt closer to the source of the Divine Feminine energy. Although I wasn't raised with religion, the little I *did* know seemed to repeat the sacred acts I'd seen in Egypt—such as Isis's magical conception of Horus, and Mary's immaculate conception of Jesus. Egypt was my access point to Source and my unique divine lineage.

Upon moving to France, I asked Thoth and Isis about the connection between Egypt and France. Had Mary Magdalene come over to France on a boat on the Mediterranean? Why had so many Mary Magdalene chapels been built on ancient temples dedicated to Isis? The response I received from the guides was yes, initiates had trained in Egypt, including Mary Magdalene, and they'd carried love teachings across the Mediterranean to France.

However, that wasn't all. This journey was also reflected in the cosmos. Isis showed me a galactic doorway, a lost temple of Isis off the coast of Saintes-Maries-de-la-Mer, where the soul would prepare for an incarnation, choosing gifts, talents, and the highest purpose of a lifetime. From this plinth of higher heart knowledge many ambassadors of love incarnated in Egypt and France to share their teachings. This illuminated for me a deeper understanding of why many lightworkers are drawn to journey to the sacred sites of Egypt and France.

My soul's journey, which brought me to France, was a doorway that required healing. I needed to move from the higher consciousness wisdom of the upper chakras, which I had developed through my connection with Thoth (infinite knowledge), to open my heart and Isis (love) wings even more. To become an embodiment of heart wisdom. I started leading groups in France. The magic continued, for the Magdalenes (a group of love beings including Anna, Isis, Mary Magdalene, the Black Madonna, and many galactic beings) would make appearances in the channelings that we undertook. I distinctly remember that the Magdalene Molecule Code (more on this code later) stepped forward during a rainy day by Saint-Maximin-la-Sainte-Baume, a sacred mountain dedicated to Mary Magdalene.

Given that I was steeped in my advanced spiritual partnership with Thoth, I didn't give these beautiful and infrequent handful of visits from the Magdalenes too much attention. In 2016, Thoth and I brought in the phenomenal body of work Divine Light Activation, which is all about embodying your light being self, and is a true game changer.

For almost eight years I didn't have the call to go back to Egypt. Then I got the message to bring a group of adepts, who had studied intensively with Thoth and the council, to Egypt for a Magdalene journey. *Magdalene* is a title meaning "a level of adeptness with energy, an ambassador of love." The guidance was very clear—we were not to go back to Egypt for more initiations, we were to go back as adepts. In 2020, we celebrated my fiftieth birthday in Egypt with divine family, a council of Divine Light Activation graduates. The Magdalene Codes began emerging more fully during this journey.

The Ecstatic Bliss Code of Love was downloaded at Hathor's temple in Dendera and the Magic of Love Code at Abydos. On February 17, 2020, while sailing on the Nile, I downloaded this first written message about the Magdalene Codes of Love body of work.

A Message from Thoth and Isis
Scribed on 2/17/20 in Egypt

Hello Dear Ones, this is Thoth with Isis, speaking on behalf of the Magdalene Midwives Council of which we are a part. The Love Conception refers to the energy of creation being resurrected for a grand purpose of the becoming. It is not only what you have already experienced as individuals that is key to this awakening, it is also that which you are designed to bring forward on this Earth plane in cocreation with others, in oneness that inspires next-level contribution and connection. The Love Conception is a formula (we are looking for a better word but for now we will use this one) of restoring the original divine gene. The divine gene is the molecular consciousness that is coherent and compatible with Source, as Source, and flowing with Source. This divine gene is such that when it is active it enables you to stream more divine energy and love in to every "now-moment."

You can think of the divine gene as a way of becoming a very concentrated liquid point of Source energy. This potent, luminous embodied divinity facilitates an even greater awakening of higher consciousness. You are divine Source. You are awakened Source. You are conscious light. The divine gene creates synergy between your bipedal form and you as Source so you become one with love, an emanation of the light, and a fountain of love; it aligns you to be love.

The love we are referring to here is not the emotion alone. It's divine love, a state where you are in communion with the highest awakened consciousness. Each time you have felt the presence and the absence of love, you can imagine that it has been a placeholder for the divine gene to be returned to the Earth Star. It's been hidden in every moment of falling in love, being in love, longing for love, grieving for love, feeling separate from love. This is all a part of the return to love. This Love Conception of divine love, from our perspective, is the most aligned consciousness that is ready to come to Earth, and now is the time.

Many of you have been on the path of awakening for eons. You have created beautiful things with light. This is important. Much has already been downloaded about the energies of light, and all that can be conceived from light. Now it is time for love.

Love Conception refers to many things and is multidimensional, which is why the Codes of Love are coming forward at this time. The Codes of Love are simultaneously a being of love and a pathway to awakening. The path has been consecrated, and we would step aside at this time. Know that each chapter, each Magdalene Code, is from a unique council of love.

ALL IS LOVE, AND WE ARE ALL,
THOTH, ISIS, AND THE MAGDALENE MIDWIVES

Entering into the Magdalene Codes

Upon returning to France from Egypt, we had our first lockdown. During the next nine months I continued to scribe the codes with the Magdalenes. On 11/11/2020 the Magdalenes and I offered them to the first group. The Magdalenes shared more about the purpose of the codes: to open the heart and turn on the love body in order to exponentially broadcast all the light we lightworkers embody. They revealed that the codes are designed to facilitate a state of being re-Sourced (to be connected to Source with overflowing resources) and to accelerate manifestation in an entirely new way, to actualize resources to champion our soul's mission and life's purpose. The Magdalenes transmitted how the codes assist us in receiving more without doing more. They burst the lies of illusion that posit that overworking, pushing, and all the do, do, do is what creates results. The codes break the illusion lie that when one form of abundance goes up, another goes down, like money increasing as free time decreases.

We put out the call for the inaugural group to gather, and thirty-two incredible souls showed up. I began that program burnt out, with my masculine energy unbalanced. My business was doing amazingly well, and I was tired. I am a stickler for walking my talk, and knew that this body of work would be transformational for those joining—and for me as well. However, I didn't realize the full extent of the new wave of higher consciousness the Magdalenes were bringing (and continue to bring) into my life and the ripple effect that would continue to have for me personally and in leading a global movement based on love and inner radiance.

For example, I had received the guidance a few years earlier that I would have a seven-figure business working three days a week, which at the time felt unrealistic. I was plugged into my business seven days a week, checking email or Facebook every day, all the time. As much as I wanted to make the change to have more analog days, and develop other areas of my life in addition to my already thriving mission, I wasn't following through with the new habits I needed to practice to make this happen. Until, that is, I had the support of the Magdalene Codes, where I easily shifted to four-day workweeks, recapturing one day a week for other things. Fast-forward until now, where the original vision is a reality.

The results that clients in the program created were also extraordinary and always unique to what the individual's mission required and what mattered most to them. On the money side of things, magic was afoot. One client received $400,000 in passive and unexpected income over a two-month period. Another received an unexpected $7,000 tax refund and was able to pay off past expenditures. One client inherited multimillions on the eve that we dove into the Yummy Money Code. For others, increasing health and relationships were top priority, which they created, going from low energy to becoming radiant and pain free. Other clients grew their businesses to reach more clients with sold-out programs, speaking opportunities, and a newfound joy of being even more visible—and much more.

As you enter into the Magdalene Codes and use this manifestation deck, know that what you actualize will be connected to what matters most to your mission and what you are aligned with. The stars are the limit, and all is possible. Welcome home, beloved of Isis and Nephthys, Magdalene adept. Enjoy being the manifestation master you truly are. I'm sending you love and blessings for your mission in this lifetime. May you create the resources that will deeply nourish and support your highest contribution to the evolution in consciousness. It takes all of us. Let's evolve consciousness together.

WITH A MAGDALENE HEART,
DANIELLE

A NEW PARADIGM OF MANIFESTING

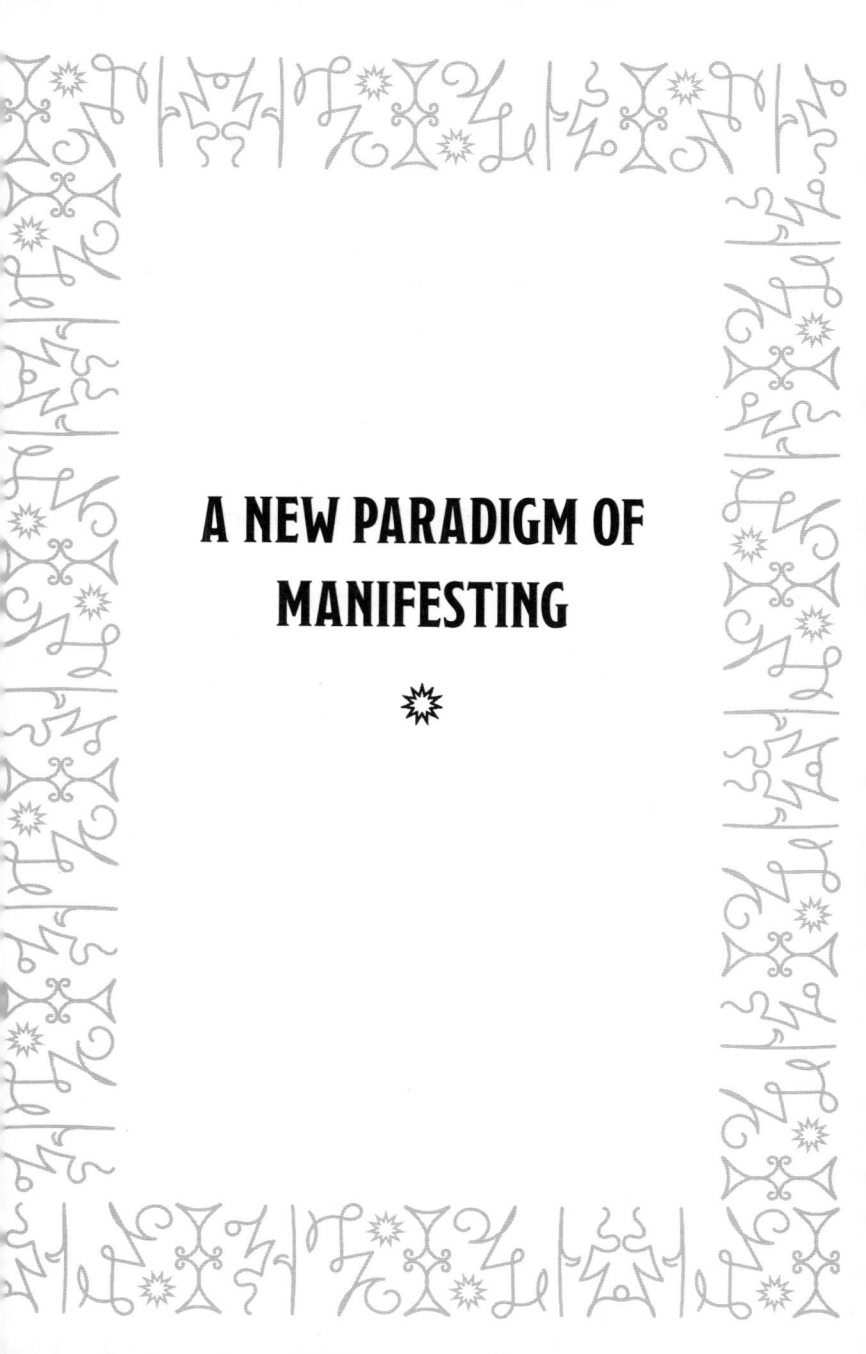

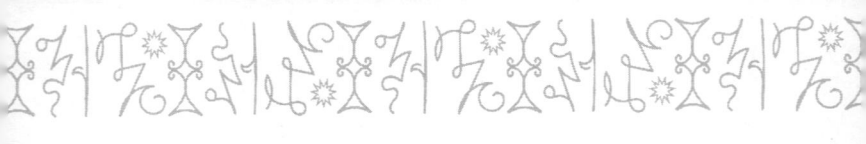

Meet the Magdalenes

Hello, dear one, we are the Magdalene Midwives from the Fully Realized divine-verse moving into the forefront of this divine transmission. We are delighted you have found your way to this Multi-D Abundance manifestation deck. As we begin our journey together, we would like to introduce ourselves. We are Magdalenes past, present, and future. The word *Magdalene* is primarily associated with Mary Magdalene and feminine love beings. However, we are a council of Divine Feminine *and* Divine Masculine beings of love; ascended masters in sacred union. Our solar feminine beings are beings such as Sekhmet; our lunar masculine beings include beings such as Ptah. Our council also includes Mary Magdalene and Yeshua, Isis and Osiris, Thoth and Seshat, and many galactic Magdalenes from beyond the central sun, including the Hathors, Nut, Nephthys, and more. We have brought forward the Magdalene Codes of Love in response to your asking and your calling, for you—beloved, be-loved—are also Magdalene.

Magdalene as a title means an adept with energy. You are here to remember and accelerate your adeptness in creating your deepest desires utilizing one of the most untapped resources on the Earth Star, which is divine love. As a Magdalene, you are a being of love, just as we the Magdalene Midwives* are a council of beings of love in light—we reside in the nonphysical planes. You are in form, multidimensional, and reside in both the physical plane and the energy planes. You have taken a physical body but you also have an energetic love and abundance body.

Our primary purpose of coming together is to cocreate Love Conceptions. Love Conceptions are also known as creations, manifestations, projects, and abundance. When conceived from love as a Magdalene, these conceptions exist in physical form and have a multidimensional, energetic love body. Manifesting with the Magdalene Codes is a process of reclaiming and accelerating your capacity to manifest in wholeness, in the new vibration of "All is well, now what?" This emanates from a deep knowing—an understanding that what is required now is different from what was required even a few short years ago.

You know what it was like in the old paradigm. Here you created from lack, from an unbalanced masculine energy of overthinking, overdoing, and a lot of action based on the fear of not being enough or not having enough. This way of operating most likely felt off to you. You've known that there is a better way. The old form of creating from scarcity, separation, fear, doubt, and worry is outdated.

The new paradigm of unity consciousness—creating from and as love—is the name of the game. This requires a recalibration of your system as an ambassador of love, a creator being. It necessitates a reclaiming of your adeptness to create using

---

*To forge a deeper connection with the Magdalenes, see our What's Next section to access your complimentary Meet the Magdalenes Channeled Guided Meditation.

multidimensional energy. As well, it requires a capacity on your part to architect conducive energetic environments. In these, your creations, your Love Conceptions, will have a vessel or energy container by which to cross the threshold from energy into form. These vessels—energetic environments, vortexes, vessels, and sacred geometry containers—are what you will create in the card spreads. Here Love Conceptions are nourished in order to take form.

This advanced manifestation technique is easy to apply and creates rapid results on the physical plane.

Support Your Mission with Multi-D Abundance and the Four Resource Codes

In order to create your deepest desires, which include the fulfillment of your mission on Earth and the deep down, to-the-bone fulfillment that comes with that, you require resources. You require abundance. Your mission requires abundance. We have chosen four resources because they touch most of you. They are what we call Yummy Money, Sublime Time, Divine Relationships, and Radiant Energy. These four resource codes are aspects of your multidimensional abundance body. Both your Multi-D Abundance body and your Magdalene Love Body recognize that wealth and abundance are actually multidimensional and unique to you and your mission.

What your particular life path requires in each and every now moment is absolutely tailored to you. Multi-D Abundance is what matters most to you and you are aligned with in your mission. This is a demarcation point, for it reflects the move from a blanket approach of manifestation to one that recognizes the bespoke, personal nature of your unique path in this lifetime. One of the foundational tenets of this practice is the spiritual truth that it is no longer necessary to grow one resource at the expense of another. For example: Your time goes up and your money goes down. Your relationships get juicier, or you have more of them, and then your energy is zapped. These are up/down resources and a function of duality. They represent the old paradigm that you are leaving behind.

Utilizing unity consciousness, you will create wholeness from wholeness instead.

The Codes Are Universal Principles to Manifest in Sacred Union

As a Magdalene conceiving the Love Conceptions that are your manifestations, you are re-Sourced. In this state you are overflowing as a creator love being. Each of the codes is a state of being or truth that you operate from, similar to a code of honor, a guideline, principle, or standard that you live by. You can think of them as your personal guidebook for manifesting in the new paradigm.

The Magdalene Codes are universal principles that remind your system that as a creator being conceiving your day—for your day is also a manifestation—you create from the energy of love as a being of love. These creations of yours have a Divine Masculine aspect and a Divine Feminine aspect that come into sacred union to be created into form, like the Divine Child.

In this card deck you will find two images for each of the twenty Codes of Love. You will find a *key* glyph (a *masculine* emanation of the Code of Love) and a *hologram* glyph (a *feminine* emanation of the Code of Love). A glyph is a sacred geometry image—a visual emanation of the code. The fact that we have two types recognizes the sacred union that resides within these two aspects in wholeness. As such, each code is a unified love being that you can invite to be a part of your manifestation council to support your creations to come into form.

The union of the masculine and feminine in this way is one of the primary principles of this card deck and is also what makes it unique. What also makes this deck exceptional is that it is a manifestation deck. The images of the codes in your card spreads create an energy vortex that is like a womb in which your creations develop to be birthed and come into full fruition. This has been one of the missing links in your practice of manifestation: you haven't been reminded that in order to create with energy, the energy needs a place in which to land. It needs a home, vessel, container, a womb space in which to grow. This is what we mean by an energy vortex.

Again, this is what the card spreads provide.

It's also important to keep in mind that what you're manifesting is a love being. Rather than thinking that you're actualizing an inanimate object, you're midwifing a *being*. Your Love Conceptions are beings of love—alive, dynamic, ever-evolving, and ever-expanding.

Let's summarize what we've covered. We have introduced ourselves as Magdalene Midwives—past, present, and future—from the Fully Realized divine-verse, which resides in a state of sacred union. We have illuminated our mission to partner with you from a place of equanimity and equality, from a place of

Meet the Magdalenes 7

love being to love being. We do this to usher in the new paradigm of manifestation.

We have shared that the Magdalene Codes of Love are universal principles that guide you to live in unity consciousness. They are also, as you've learned, Magdalene Love Beings. There is a feminine Magdalene being and a masculine Magdalene being for each of the twenty Codes of Love. We also have four Magdalene beings that are resource codes, with a single image in sacred union. In total, we have forty-four cards that you will use in your manifestation practice.

As a Magdalene, which you also are, you create abundance through love. Abundance in the new paradigm is multidimensional, and as such, it's meant to grow in simultaneity. From our experience of working with thousands of you, we've noticed a pattern that is frequently at play: your abundance will reach a ceiling, or you will unconsciously put on the brakes. Thus you can also look at the Magdalene Code deck as an upper-limit buster, a crossing of the threshold around those perceived blocks—those upper limits where you've manifested a portion of your desires but not 100 percent of them.

We've also spoken about the card deck spreads creating energy vortexes or womb space for your creations or your love beings to come into form.

We are delighted that you have found your way to this deck, and we look forward to being a part of your manifestation council!

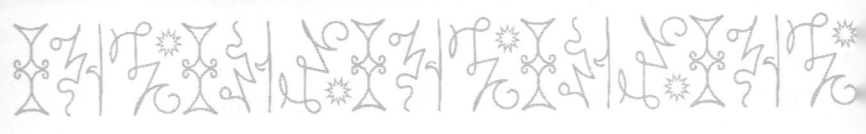

Five Spiritual Truths of 5D Manifesting as a Magdalene

Now that we've transmitted the big picture of the new paradigm of manifesting and the Magdalene Codes, let's go deeper into the five principles of multidimensional (multi-D) manifesting, including 5D and beyond. These are universal principles—spiritual truths that simultaneously provide a shift in perception and assist you in deepening your alignment with the new paradigm.

One: Your Creations Are Beings of Light

There are many of what we call "illusion lies" that represent the old paradigm of separation consciousness and, as such, are on their way out. The first illusion lie that we would bust is that your creations are inanimate 3D objects. Again (and we are repeating this to underscore its importance), the spiritual truth is that your creations are beings of light: alive, dynamic, ensouled energies. This body of work, the Magdalene Codes, and the extensions of the card deck, guidebook, and program is a multidimensional being of light. The home that you live in is a being of light. Your resources such as money, time, relationships, and energy are beings of light.

When you make this perceptual shift you amplify your capacity to partner with your manifestations in ways that are highly magnetic and extraordinary. In so doing you are acknowledging that your manifestations have a purpose, innate intelligence, and support. In this new territory of unity consciousness versus separation consciousness, the Divine expands through love, cocreation, harmony, joy, and abundance.

The source of all of your manifestations is Source. Source is infinite; therefore, there is an infinite supply of the source of your creations that is available to you to connect to as you are creating resources. Money is a being that is connected to the infinite supply of money, time is a being that is connected to all of time, relationships are a being that is connected to the source of all relationships. Money often comes to you through other people; however, the origin of that money is Source. These individuals are not your source. Source is your source. Realizing that the resources you have in your pool of abundance are not fixed and finite but alive and connected to the infinite supply allows you to receive more fully and easily. In this you midwife your own manifestations through love. Midwifing manifestations is perhaps a new concept, which brings us to the next universal truth.

Two: All That There Is Exists in Each and Every Moment

It can feel daunting when you approach your manifestations, as if all the responsibility for making them happen is on your shoulders and you have to create something out of thin air. The primary tenet of separation consciousness is that something is missing and often broken that needs to be fixed. Creating from this place of lack perpetuates the old paradigm of what is called "lack consciousness." Creating from the energy of surplus not only feels better to your system, it also accelerates your manifestations.

If you remember the universal truth that all that there is exists in each and every moment, you remind your system of surplus, of abundance as a birthright, as a given. It currently exists in an energetic form in the higher planes. As well, the correlating cooperative components already exist on the physical plane. For it to come into form, you simply need to come into vibrational proximity to it.

Let's say you deeply desire to actualize a loving romantic partnership. The individual you desire already exists; it's not that they are being born right now and have to be created from scratch. Let's say you are thirty, fifty, or seventy. Your partner is not only in energy form, they are already on the planet. Again, you are simply not in vibrational proximity with them. This is the same with your desires and your Multi-D Abundance projects, creations, and manifestations to be. If you have the desire to actualize them, they already exist. They are beings of light in light and it's a joy to bring them from energy forms into energy *in* form.

This spiritual truth quickly shifts you from lack consciousness, for you recognize that what you desire is also seeking you. In this there is not any kind of separation—this is an illusion lie. This shifting of your consciousness aligns you with the higher principles of "This or something better," for in this scenario, manifestation is based on an amplification of love and life for all, and honors free will and conscious choice. You can already commune and talk with the being of light that is your home, or the being that represents your financial freedom, or that of your thriving career, or that of a loving relationship. You acknowledge that all of these are in the form of energy, which, again, has yet to be fully nourished and cultivated in order to come into form. As well, you acknowledge that the elements necessary to manifest them into form already exist on the physical plane. As such, most of them are associated with the four resource codes of Yummy Money, Sublime Time, Divine Relationships, and Radiant Energy.

Three: Expand Your Horizontal Love Body to Receive More Without Doing More

The Magdalene Codes expand your capacity to receive more without doing more. How does this work? You pass approximately two-thirds of your day with your body in a vertical position standing or sitting; your spinal column is vertical. This verticality is connected to your light, to the Divine Masculine.

The horizontal plane, on the other hand, represents your energetic width, breadth, reach, and receptive capacities. If you hold your arms out to the left and right of your body, this is your horizontal plane, which does not end at your fingertips. Your horizontal energy body is connected to your heart center, and to how much love you have running in your system. Love is one of the most inclusive energies there is and is a highly receptive vibration. It is the new paradigm of unity consciousness and it's associated with the chakra that you and the Earth Star are increasingly embodying.

The Magdalene Codes assist your horizontal plane and energy body—your horizontal love body—to widen and be more receptive so that your actualizations have a wider surface area to connect with you. When you lie down, your spinal column is in a horizontal position. You become wider where your physical body takes up a wider surface area.

The superpower of the Magdalene Manifester is utilizing the often overlooked, ignored, and forgotten Divine Feminine capacities of manifesting that include creating in the dreamtime, resting, being, and physicalizing through the vibrational matching of frequencies. The Magdalene Codes—especially when you create card spreads before you go to sleep, take a nap, or lie down in a meditative position (all of which feature your body in a horizontal position)—directly assist you in putting out a vibrational signal on the nonphysical plane that connects to the source of whatever resource you are drawing into your life. Again, in this we are specifically working with Yummy Money, Sublime Time, Divine Relationships, and Radiant Energy.

The source of all these resources is always Source and comes to you through individuals, experiences, and opportunities. The Magdalene Codes assist you in amplifying your horizontal energy field with a wider broadcast signal that makes you even more receptive and magnetic to the Multi-D Abundance that your divine mission requires. This assists you to receive more without doing more because you have a wider surface area in which to receive abundance. In other words, you're not trying to receive the ocean in the thimble of a contracted energy body or into the needle of a shutdown energy body.

Width is one of the dimensions of 3D (height, width, and

depth), which, when expanded, is key to actualizing in the physical plane while also accessing dimensions beyond 3D. Lightworkers have often developed and increased their verticality, thereby expanding the height of their energetic field. What lightworkers require now is love. This book, *Magdalene Manifestation Cards,* is our love letter to you to balance and integrate all the light that you've accumulated from being bipedal with two feet, two arms, two hands, two eyes, two ears, and a vertical spinal column. In order to apply all the light that you've been calling in and developing, more light isn't required to move the needle. What *is* required is the incorporation of the quality of love so that the light and the love are in sacred union. The masculine and feminine are in sacred union—the physical and nonphysical are in wholeness, and the result is that you are in wholeness.

The animals on your Earth Star have a horizontal spinal column. For example, horses, cats, and dogs have bodies that feature the wide horizontal plane of their backs and the shorter vertical plane of their legs. So they do have some verticality. The spinal column, the earthly and the heavenly chi, is moving in a left-right direction in horses, cats, dogs, and many animals. Your earthly and heavenly chi move in an up/down direction.

Your Magdalene Codes widen your horizontal body. To help visualize this you can sit or lie down in the middle of the floor and place the twenty hologram cards to your left and the twenty key cards to your right in a horizontal line expanding outward from your heart center. You can see how this widens your horizontal plane and bandwidth to receive more without doing more; each code is a dimension of your abundance body. You can also place the four resource cards in a horizontal plane along the front of your body to create a cross. In this, your resources are exponentiated by the horizontal plane.

When the heart is closed, your manifestations are trying to squeeze through the eye of a needle. You don't have enough receptor sites in your energy body, or you do but they're not fully lined up with the whole. You have created amazing things using the unbalanced masculine energy of doing, doing, doing, going, going, going, overthinking, overthinking, overthinking. And when you're aligned and centered you've also been using the balanced aspects of the masculine energy to create, which is your capacity to take inspired action, hold a line of sight and go directly for something you desire.

However, in the new era of higher consciousness, the feminine quality of love is what is required now.

Remember, your heart is one of the most receptive organs in the body, and opening your heart makes you a million times more magnetic, as does consciously cultivating your horizontal energy field. Working with the Magdalene cards assists you with both.

Four: Create Energy Containers to Manifest at the Speed of Love

The creation of energy containers is essential to the process of successful manifestation. This energetic secret makes all the difference between manifesting 100 percent of your desires every time and trying a bunch of things (taking action, meditating, working with a business coach) to get the desired results, making progress yet still not reaching the full realization of your targets. As you know, everything is energy, and you are most likely aware of the quantum field of infinite possibilities. The process of bringing your creations (beings of light) that are already manifested in the higher planes into form on the physical plane is one where you utilize your connection to energy.

Creating energetic containers through the glyphs of each code provides a landing pad for your creations. It is like having a net with which to catch a ball or fish. You are creating a beautiful home for your actualizations to magnetize all the cooperative components to it. This is a magical game changer and will forever elevate your practice of manifestation. We invite you to be open to embracing this love technology of creating energetic containers in order that your journey with the codes is an uplevel and fresh start in your manifestation adeptness—no matter what you have tried before that hasn't worked.

The reason this works so well is multifaceted. Let's dive into a few reasons here. Most likely you are not manifesting what you desire because unconsciously you are repelling it. The reason for this may be that you associate a cost with it. For example, you may have experienced an increase in financial abundance and a simultaneous decrease in your energy or time with loved ones. Manifesting financial abundance was associated with a cost you didn't want to incur.

You may be repelling it because, again, it may feel as if the abundance will come at a cost, or you think something you value will be diminished. If you create more abundance you may fear losing love, leaving someone behind, or being judged, or you have a fear of getting killed or ostracized. Highly sensitive lightworkers often sense the separation consciousness and slower vibrations overlaid onto things. As an example, say in the past someone who was depressed paid you money. You may have empathically felt their depression overlaid onto the money or a responsibility to change it, which felt uncomfortable. Thus, you may unconsciously avoid receiving money, because you have confounded the negative energy overlaid onto money (and there are a lot of slower vibrations projected upon money) with the actual signature energy of money, which is neutral. Thus, out of self-preservation, you avoid repeating the original scenario.*

Take a moment and tune in to see what you may be afraid of if more abundance comes into your life.

As you do so please note that the energetic container you will be creating is calibrated to be magnetic and inclusive of not only the result (more money, time, relationships, or energy), it will also provide you with optimal circumstances surrounding the shift from where you are to where you are choosing to be in ways that enhance the ecosystem of your entire abundance body.

When you create energy containers and envision that your creations are love beings, and you widen your heart and horizontal field, you become highly receptive. Your creations, which at their origin are energy in the nonphysical plane, have an energy form on the physical plane to be midwifed and grounded into. The glyphs and cards are multidimensional and holographic, creating a sacred geometry pattern that is coherent and connected to energies that your manifestations require to come into form. They are nurturing and supportive to your system as well.

Being a cocreator of the energy vortex with Source and the

---

*See the What's Next section to learn additional steps you can take to enhance your relationship with money through our channeled Yummy Money workshop (our gift to you).

Magdalene Codes allows you and the light being of your creation to be detached, neutral, and in the midwife's seat. This reclaims your feminine dynamic of receiving more without doing more.

Five: Aligned Action from the Impulse of Creation Creates Worlds

The Magdalene Codes lean heavily on the Divine Feminine ways of manifesting, for those are the ones that have often been suppressed. As the feminine ways of manifesting through energy come more online, the Divine Masculine naturally comes back into balance. As we've shared, the sacred union of the two creates the Divine Child, manifestation in wholeness. Action alone is not what creates your manifestations. If that were the case and you've been in action then you would have created what you desire already. Many who work with us are high performers, high achievers, and are no strangers to taking action, proactively and consistently. If this sounds like you, adding in the Magdalene Manifestation cards will skyrocket your results and leverage what you've already taken action upon. For after all, action is a primary reason you chose to incarnate rather than just play in the energetic realms alone.

But perhaps, like many of our clients—who in addition to being high performers are also spiritually advanced and energy savvy—the inverse is true for you and you have *not* been taking action. Rather, you have been in a holding pattern of waiting, trying to figure things out, hanging back, or being in input mode (getting another certification, listening to podcasts, asking others for what action you should take), rather than sharing your mission with others. Or maybe you've been diligently visualizing your desires or leaning *only* on energetic practices; in this case, what may move the needle for you is action and the masculine energy, so pay special attention when the key codes appear in your spreads. Most likely, like most of our clients, you have a combination of too much yin in some areas and too much yang in others. You may find that you put a lot of focus on and take a lot of action in certain areas of your Multi-D Abundance, such as working or money, while neglecting relationships and health. And vice versa: your vibrations may be amplifying feminine principles in certain places and relationships in your life, but not at all in others.

Regardless of where you are on the yin-yang spectrum of being and action, the Magdalene Codes assist you in bringing homeostasis between the two so that you may joyfully take inspired action. Energy and resources do indeed require a physical plane pathway to come into your life, so action is an important component of the whole. This action may surprise you, for it may be action that bubbles up from the impulse of creation. It may be action that emerges from your deeper awareness and Heart-Sentience.

With each card description you'll deepen into the holographic feminine glyph to recalibrate your being state and the key masculine glyph to amplify your action state. Plus, you'll tap into the essence of the code in sacred union to amplify the Divine Child creation of your manifestation as it comes into form.

You came to Earth to create in the physical realm and taking aligned action is one of the coveted ways you get to play on the Earth Star. Enjoy midwifing your manifestations for the joy of it—not from a place of need or lack but from a place of exploration and confident creating instead!

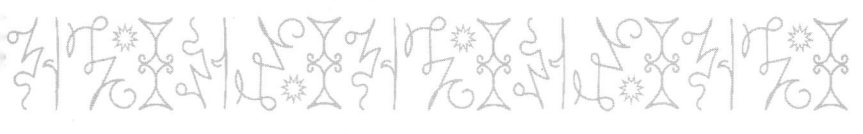

How to Use This Manifestation Deck
A Multidimensional Love Technology

You may be familiar with oracle or divination decks where you pull cards to receive guidance and direction. However, this may be the first time you are using cards as a multidimensional manifestation practice. It may be the first time you've contemplated creating energy vortexes to hold space in which your manifestations may then materialize. Although this love technology may feel new at times, it is quite easy to implement.

The codes are beings of light, and each card has a glyph (high vibrational visual representation of the code) that is multidimensional. When you pull cards from the deck they form an altar, energetic container, and energy vortex for your desire to have a home, a place to be held and embraced vibrationally by the Codes of Love. This creates a highly magnetic energy vortex that calls to it all that your desire requires to come into fruition. You may be wondering what types of manifestations you can dedicate your card spreads to. We use the words *manifestation, physicalization,* and *actualization* interchangeably. When you sit down to do a card spread with this deck—for it is primarily a manifestation deck—you're choosing to manifest or actualize something. It is important to be really clear on what the different dimensions of your desired manifestations are.

When we first talk about manifestation what may come to you is manifesting something physical like a car, home, money, job, or relationship. These external *physical* goals are perfectly clear and familiar to you, and no doubt you have a good idea what those desires are.

Getting clear on what it is that you really desire on the *soul* level can be a bit more ephemeral, nebulous, or seem almost out of reach. We want to open the possibilities of your manifestation spreads to be one of infinite possibilities. Absolutely use this card deck to manifest physical resources that contribute to and champion your soul's purpose in this lifetime and are fun and enjoyable. Also use this card deck to create altars for ways of being, for your emotional well-being, for a mood, a consistent home zone frequency that you come from, as well as to cultivate divine qualities like joy and peace. Use this manifestation deck to create peace of mind, coherence, alignment, joy, fun, and truth, to have a space to advance your path of evolution and enlightenment, and to experience connection to Source. In other words, use this manifestation deck not only to meet your physical desires, needs, and relationships, but also for your internal states and ways of being, for these are interconnected.

You desire to manifest something because of what you anticipate the beneficial results will be. For example you may associate financial freedom—having a passive income that surpasses your needs—with feeling great, secure, and having the luxury of a fair amount of free time. You associate the things, the individuals, the experiences, the states of being that you desire with various states of being. Creating altars to manifest states of being is something that you can absolutely have control over now, and making the necessary internal perception shift can be instantaneous.

You can always shift your inner state of being. When you manifest what you want, especially with the four Multi-D Abundance resource cards—Yummy Money, Sublime Time, Divine Relationships, Radiant Energy—focus not only on the Sublime Time you have or are choosing to manifest but also on how it will feel to have an abundance of time to spend in ways that light you up. And cultivate that feeling tone now, on the journey and at the destination. Cultivate the internal experience of joy, generosity, safety, or whatever you associate that money, time, relationship, or energy will create within you and who you sense you'll get to become in the process. Master your energy, unlock your preferred feeling state, tap into your future self, and experience the joys of your manifestation *now*.

Create Altars for Manifesting

Get imaginative with your focus and the purpose of these altars, manifestations, and card deck spreads. Dedicate them to your projects. For example, if you are writing a book or creating a business, create a card spread, an altar, a Magdalene Council of Love Codes that will hold your vision in an energetic container to become Fully Realized, with the mindset of this or something better.

The desire that you have may also be a desire to bring you into closer proximity with something else. For example, in her twenties your beloved divine transmitter Danielle took kundalini yoga classes when she was a massage therapist, and also massaged white tantric yoga facilitators. This all came into her life. It wasn't something she was seeking out. She started doing kundalini yoga. She also had a longtime desire to go to the Grand Canyon. There happened to be a kundalini yoga retreat not far from the Grand Canyon.

She followed these desires to go to the Grand Canyon and do the yoga retreat on one trip. She manifested these desires in and of themselves. What she wasn't anticipating is that she would meet her beloved life partner and husband, Friedemann, at the yoga camp. Sometimes the desire that you have is also positioning you to come into vibrational proximity with another experience or individual. This is where you are focused and yet you're in a state of neutrality. You're in a state of nonattachment. You're in this place of, "I'm going for this. I'm going to the Grand Canyon. I'm going to have this experience of spiritual evolution." Then when something else comes onto your path, you are open to that. You're present to that.

We invite you to primarily focus on your manifestation spreads for you, but you can also create energy vortexes for others. If they don't choose to receive them then they will just go back into the wholeness, back into the oneness. You can program your manifestation spreads and your energy vortexes so that if the energy isn't used, it goes to the Earth or it contributes to humanity or to somebody else you may not know who is asking for similar support in some way.

You can create a spread for the highest and best experience of that day by pulling a code of the Magdalene being who's going to be with you during that day, starting when you wake up in the morning. You can create a spread for a meeting, a job interview, getting into college, hiring your business manager, drawing to you aligned, perfectly matched clients, your community of friends, or like-minded individuals.

You can create Divine Relationship altars if there is some friction or noncoherence in a relationship with someone. Let's say there is some friction in your workplace; you can do a spread for the highest outcome for your coworkers. Also remember that when something doesn't manifest it may be creating something you desire even more, or leading you on a more aligned path. Being *all in* on manifesting your desires—while holding them lightly and coming from a place of neutrality—and being open to something even better materializing is a magical combination and one we can't underscore enough. Have fun with your manifesting practice, and please don't use it to beat yourself up if you create something else instead of what you were going for. Remember your Multi-D Abundance is directly tied to your mission and what matters most to you. Your creations will reflect this deeper current of truth of who you are and what resources your path in this lifetime requires.

We go into more detail about how to use these cards, and specific card spreads, in the next parts of this book.

Energy Vortexes for Internal and External Manifestations

We've gone over some different possibilities that you can create spreads for. With any manifestation, there is the journey and there is the destination. There is how you feel about the manifestation and then there is your creation of the manifestation. When you go into your Yummy Money, Sublime Time, Divine Relationships, or Radiant Energy spreads you realize your relationship with money, how you feel about money, your experience with money, beliefs about money, and your internal manifestations around money. Then there are your external manifestations with money.

Let's say you're choosing to actualize ten thousand dollars, a hundred thousand dollars, a million dollars, or whatever money target is aligned with you. There is external physicalized money in your bank account. Then there is your relationship with the money being of light and love. We would invite you, as you are creating your altars pertaining to money or any resource, to build altars and energy vortexes for both internal and external manifestations. Your inner state of being—"As above so below, as within so without"—is very important to your external manifestations. We can't emphasize this enough.

For those of you who love to play in your inner world and the being state, you may have a lot of feminine energy and be very receptive. Given this, we invite you to take fierce action, to get your hands in the clay, to actualize. This is not about creating altars and then not acting as the action presents itself. If we go back to the example of Danielle manifesting being in vibrational proximity with her beloved, there was a lot of action that went into that. She took yoga classes, said yes to traveling to the Grand Canyon, booked her plane ticket, packed her clothes . . . you get the idea.

In this she encountered the physical pathway, red carpet, or conveyor belt of now-moments that lined up in order that she meet her beloved, and saying yes and saying no along the way. As part of their love story, she and Friedemann spent the week together as friends and getting to know each other. Then there was a series of synchronicities where both of their respective flights were delayed an extra eighteen hours, giving them a very important window of time together. At face value, the flights being delayed and canceled were undesirable experiences. However, this turn of events created the ensuing transition in Danielle's relationship with Friedemann wherein it went from friendship to love with a beautiful life partner.

This is also why we focus on Sublime Time—your multidimensional now-moments are essential as you're actualizing what it is you desire. There is the reality of time, of twenty-four hours a day, then there is your experience of time. You have a relationship with time. Maybe your relationship in the past has been that you don't have enough time. There is a sense of more things to do than you have time to do them in or there just may not be this really lush, relaxed relationship with time.

You can shift that lack-based perspective into a deeper spiritual truth that you always have more than enough time. You have an abundance of time. There's not a lack of time. There is divine timing. Time is malleable. Time is expansive. Time is multidimensional. You can have the beliefs of knowing that you have a surplus of time, that everything gets done within the time that you have for it. Everything gets done easily and doesn't have to be done by you alone. Things are lining up in a way that constitutes the shortest and fastest path; much of this comes to you while you sleep and thus doesn't take extra time from your day.

Here is an example of the kind and degree of shift you might expect. Under the old paradigm, when you got stuck in traffic, let's say, you may have felt angry and frustrated, causing slower vibrations to arise. Under the new paradigm, in the same circumstance, you might rejoice, saying, "Wow, this is cool," because being "stuck" gives you the time and space to listen to your favorite podcast, or it gives you the beautiful experience of singing along with the music on the radio, getting a special download, or maybe enjoying a chat with a friend.

There is a whole way of being in a relationship with multidimensional time that you will experience as you become more multidimensional yourself. In this, you'll be operating in more dimensions and timelines (which we go into in the Magdalene Codes of Love program and Divine Light Activation program; learn more about this in the What's Next section). You'll be operating and utilizing your nonphysical energy to connect to other nonphysical energies that then speed up your manifestation process quite a bit. Yet if you are cranky, frustrated, exhausted, burnt out, overworked, feeling over-responsible, oversensitive, and taking on everybody's stuff in the now-moment, your inner relationship to time, which is also in the now-moment, can use some enhancement.

You can create altars around this as well. The energy created will ripple out to your relationship with Radiant Energy, your body, and your health. It will ripple out to your Divine Relationships with others, too. If you find yourself in a space of friction, lack, duality, or noncoherence in your relationship with yourself or others, create altars to switch up the energy as needed.

Come Have Tea with Us: You Are Invited into Sacred Space

As we gather for the card spreads, we would invite you to simultaneously recognize that when you choose to do a card spread you have an opportunity to meet with the Magdalene Council about the Love Conception you are creating. We will provide energy and guidance through the images, affirmations, descriptions, and our direct relationship with you. This is the divination, or the oracular aspect of the deck, and you can experience it in such a way it's like having tea with us. Take a moment to be, to be. Part of the way that the masculine and the feminine come back into sacred union is through amplification or a raising of the feminine, the being state, the receptive state.

There is the divination aspect to the card deck, or the oracle aspect to the card deck. In this, you're hanging out with your manifestation team of Magdalenes in the codes that you draw, and you receive aha moments and guidance from your higher self and from us. As we've shared, the codes also enable the creation of an energy vortex, container, womb, or vessel to magnetize all that the manifestation requires. They allow for a sacred geometry form to cross the threshold from energy into what you would call "matter," or the physical dimension to go from nonphysical to physical, with the nonphysical energy being in sacred union with the physical energy. This is another way to look at this masculine-feminine-creation dance. Right now, all that you desire and require in your Love Conceptions and manifestations already exists in the higher planes. It's already in energy form. You have the divine desire to actualize something that matters to you and your mission and it's yours to be, do, and have in alignment with the highest good of all. It already exists in the nonphysical plane. It's already done.

How is it that you come into vibrational proximity to that which exists in the nonphysical and bring it into the physical form? The Magdalene Codes help you do just that, because you create an energetic sacred geometry field with the glyphs. The images of the codes become a natural home for your manifestations to come into physical form. Just like your Ka body, your energy body, and your physical body are connected, so is your energy body connected to your manifestations. See you in the codes!

CARD DESCRIPTIONS

The first part of this guidebook houses the descriptions of each of the cards and discusses how to apply them. We've also included short explanations and keywords on the cards for ease of use. A magical aspect of card decks is that the cards stand on their own and can be rearranged and used in a nonlinear, intuitive, and organic way. The order of the codes in the guidebook reflects the order in which the codes were downloaded. You may feel called to dive right into creating manifestation spreads and working directly with the cards in ways that feel the most aligned with you.

ABOUT THE HIGH VIBRATIONAL GLYPHS ON THE CARDS

The Magdalene Codes have chosen to be expressed in high vibrational art, energy-infused visual images, or glyphs. This forty-four card deck includes a total of twenty-four Magdalene Codes. Four of these are resource codes—Yummy Money, Sublime Time, Divine Relationships, and Radiant Energy—with one card each. The remaining twenty codes are Codes of Love, with two cards per each code for a total of forty cards. As we've mentioned, each Code of Love has two images or glyphs: one key glyph and one hologram glyph. You can think of the *key* glyphs as an active external energy that opens energy in your system and your creations, allowing them to become physicalized. The *hologram* glyph encourages an internal focus and being state, where every line includes the whole. We often speak of the hologram glyphs as relating to the Divine Feminine principles of manifesting and the key glyphs relating to the Divine Masculine principles of manifesting; however, the codes and your creations are in sacred union with Source.

On each card you will see a small symbol before the caption that indicates whether it is a resource, key, or hologram code. The resource code symbol looks like a diamond, representing the four resources of Yummy Money, Sublime Time, Divine Relationships, and Radiant Energy. The key code has a symbol of a key on it. The hologram has a symbol of a sphere on the inside, with two halves of the sphere on the outside of the circle. What are some of the distinctions between the key glyph and

Resource Code Symbol

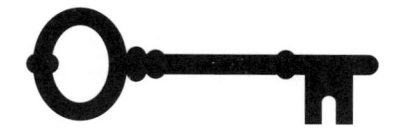

Key Code Symbol

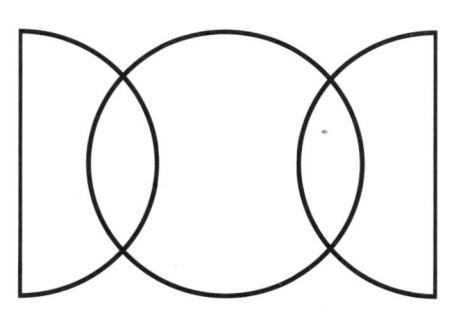

Hologram Code Symbol

the hologram glyph? You can often visually distinguish the key glyph as being more of a singular symbol, and the hologram glyph as being more of a sphere or sacred geometry pattern. The hologram has the key within it, like a fractal or an abstract or lines of the hologram. Manifesting is a process of fractal coherence wherein each line of the hologram is connected to the whole and repeats in a coherent manner. This is like the branches on a tree that repeat in fractal patterns as they grow, or yin existing within yang and vice versa.

Enjoy steeping and basking in the energies of the sacred geometry symbols and energy emanations of the Magdalene Codes.

Four Resource Codes

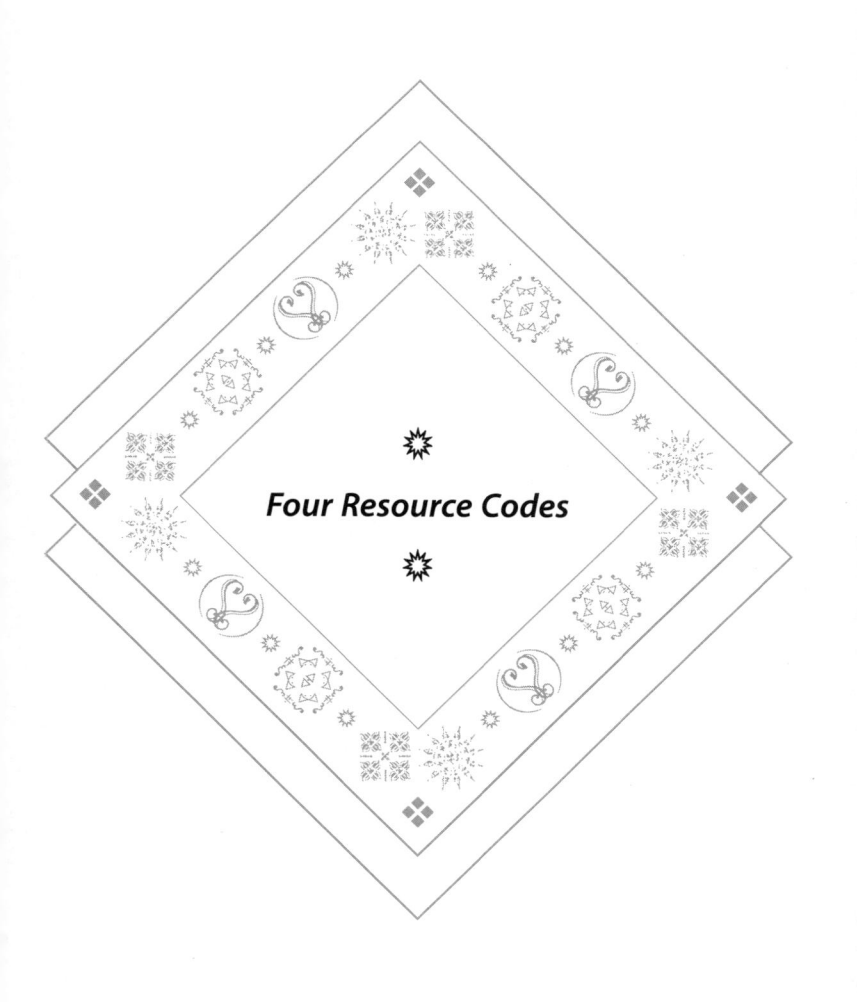

1
Yummy Money

"All money is yummy."

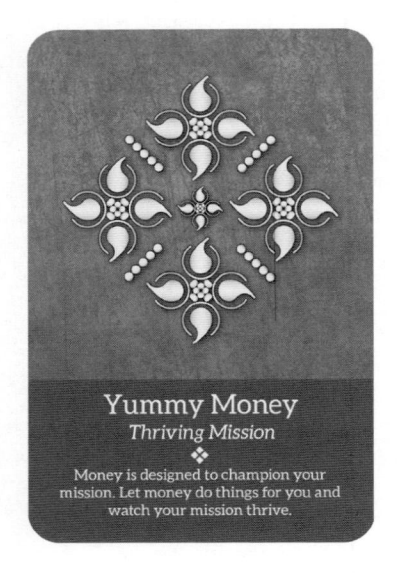

Yummy Money
Thriving Mission

Money is designed to champion your mission. Let money do things for you and watch your mission thrive.

This resource code supports you to be in the energy of "As above so below, as within so without" in regards to money—to simultaneously be uber-aligned, coherent, clear, and empowered in your internal relationship with money and also be adept in your external creation of it. Money is a part of your life for the duration of your life. The Yummy Money Code guides you as you transcend generations of turmoil around the topic of money and in creating a new legacy with money based on love, partnership, and cocreation.

Creating money is an act of self-love. It's an act of being a leader in the evolution of consciousness. You can be an even greater contribution when your money is thriving, imbued with love and the birthright of abundance. Money is a spiritual frontier. It's a way of getting your hands in the clay as a creator being. Upgrading your relationship with money to be yummy as well as externally creating it is one of the best investments of your time and energy you can make in your spiritual evolution. Oodles of untapped expansion rest in dormant repose within the topic of money, both the potential to expand your money abundance and to elevate your consciousness. Activate this divine potential. Be on the leading wave of consciousness as you craft your multi-D Yummy Money resources and relationship.

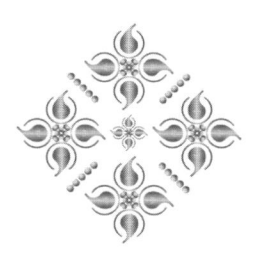

YUMMY MONEY RESOURCE
Thriving Mission

❖

> Money is designed to champion your mission. Let money do things for you and watch your mission thrive.

There is a new paradigm of money with an evolved higher purpose. When you draw this card you are invited to update your internal relationship with money to be one that is yummy—to shift from stress, worry, lack, and scarcity into abundance, cocreation, and partnership. Money is a being of love, and the resource code of Yummy Money is a being of love that connects your manifestation projects to the money being and to the source of all money, which is Source.

The new paradigm of money is based on equality and cocreation. The higher purpose of money is to create more life and abundance for all rather than the limitations of the old paradigm of money, wherein it was based on lack, or not being or having enough in a win/lose environment. The new multidimensional money paradigm is where your individual abundance circulates love in your life, family, community, and the globe. Your well-being and what is good for you is good for others, too.

Your thriving mission requires money. The Yummy Money Code encourages you to create a brand-new relationship with the energy of money as a partner who champions your purpose. Allow the life-enhancing, purpose-championing energy of money to buoy your mission, support you, and do great things for you. When you pull this card look within and ask how money can support you and your mission. What could money do for you? Perhaps your Heart-Sentience guides you to add a transformative Divine Relationship to your life, like a mentor, team member, or personal assistant to handle tasks that take you out of your zone of genius. Maybe you need to increase the flow of your money by moving or circulating it in your financial containers. Under this scenario you might raise your prices, pay off past expenditures, or have your money work for you through various investments.

When this resource code is drawn or you consciously choose to do a Yummy Money spread by building a manifestation altar, or creating a container for Yummy Money, you are also reconciling much deeper limitations of the old paradigm. For example, if you associate money in the physical plane with masculine energy and you have unresolved issues with your father or other men, you may have overlaid this onto your relationship with money. Or if you associate money with the feminine in the nonphysical plane and you have trust or abandonment issues with your mother or other women, you may repress the feminine ways of receiving and find yourself working way too hard for money. Allow this sacred union code to restore the sacred union with the feminine and masculine energies within and without. Forge a new partnership with Yummy Money that is current. "Currency" involves being current with who it is that you've become. *Currency* is also a word used to represent financial resources. Money is money. Money is yummy.

APPLICATION

When you receive, have, circulate, or interact with money in any form we invite you to bring the word *yummy* into your awareness. Say *yummy* out loud. Make a sound like *mmmm,* just like you might after eating something especially yummy. There is a vibration of the *mmms* in *money* and *yummy* that uplifts your frequency and supercharges your money Love Conceptions.

2
Sublime Time

"All time is sublime."

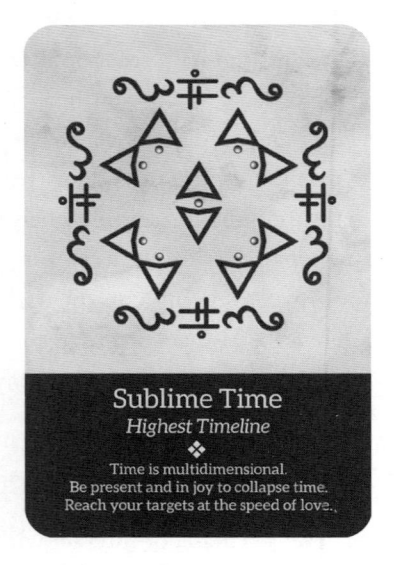

Sublime Time
Highest Timeline

Time is multidimensional.
Be present and in joy to collapse time.
Reach your targets at the speed of love.

There is a new paradigm of time in unity consciousness. The Sublime Time Code, like love, moves at a high speed. Time as a frequency is very rapid and is accelerating in velocity. Time is now, time is multidimensional. Time is a being of light.

Time is one of the resources—like money, relationships, and energy—that spans your entire life and touches all now-moments. In the old paradigm you may have experienced a lack of time and unconsciously perpetuated this by repeatedly saying things like "I don't have enough time to get everything done" or "I don't have time for that." There can be a poverty consciousness around time, as well as an overlay of the idea that you have good times and bad times, fun times and hard times.

Sublime Time is a particular being of light connected to the new paradigm of time, the being of light of time, and the source of all time, which is Source. With the Magdalene of Sublime Time, time is sublime—sublime as in enjoyable, pleasurable, joyful, ecstatic, lush, and nourishing. There is a restoration of all now-moments being in right relationship to the totality of all now, in such a way that no matter what you're up to (being or doing), your system is nourished and you're tapped into multidimensional Sublime Time.

Linear time is a construct and it's useful until it's not. Multidimensional time, on the other hand, is beyond time and space. Having the being of light that is Sublime Time join your creation Love Conceptions and manifestation containers is a gift. It accelerates the speed at which your creations come into form. With multidimensional time you can imagine that time is stacked on top of itself like in a vertical column that then is spread out over a horizontal column of now-moments. Like kundalini energy moves both vertically and horizontally, multidimensional time moves and grows in a dynamic spiral. The power to choose and to create resides within this now-moment. Sublime Time is the sacred union of how you feel in each now-moment, the experience of the external creation of time.

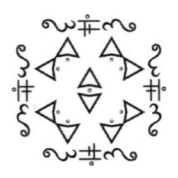

SUBLIME TIME RESOURCE
Highest Timeline

❖

> Time is multidimensional. Be present and in joy to collapse time. Reach your targets at the speed of love.

Sublime Time connects you with your highest timeline, which spans dimensions. You are physically located on the Earth, and you also have other lifetimes—past, future, or parallel lifetimes on Earth and off-planet. Sublime Time brings the gifts of all lifetimes into the potency of the now-moment to be in a state of coherence and alignment. It recalibrates your system to the spiritual truth that this now-moment is as good as any other now-moment. As you embrace this truth you experience a deep sense of relief and you recapture time from inefficient uses of your energy, such as resisting the now-moment or the emotional ups and downs that come from this resistance. Imagine how much more time you have when you stop judging your experience and start being present with it from a place of joy.

When the Sublime Time card comes into your manifestation container a treasure chest of unused units of time is available to you. You can think of this like vacation days that you may have accumulated at your job that you haven't taken. This accumulated treasure chest of time is unlocked with this code so that your project is buoyed with Sublime Time and sublime timing. Miraculous things happen quickly. Others pitch in. The feeling tone of your project is that there is always *plenty* of time. There is an overflow or a surplus in the treasure chest of time. When a lack of time, just like a lack of money, is no longer an excuse for you to hold back from creating what it is that you truly desire, your Multi-D Abundance starts to rise to the surface.

When the Sublime Time Code steps forward and you're very present in the now-moment, in the multidimensional now, multiple things happen very quickly or simultaneously. You can be focused on an activity—for example, right now you're reading this. While you're very present with this guidebook, other aspects of your abundance are moving forward in multidimensional time. This code is an anchor, magnet, or beacon that's putting out the request to the universe to line optimal experiences up for you so that things work out for the highest and best good of all.

The core elements or principles of Sublime Time are that the new paradigm of time and the being of light that's associated with time is eternal, and that there's an abundance of time. You are an eternal being and your projects have a ripening process, a divine timing gestation period. At times you may be pushing yourself harder and harder to try to get things to happen faster and faster. This actually creates fatigue, overwork, and has the opposite effect of Sublime Time. You will still take action toward your dreams, and there will be high intensity push times like when the baby is ready to come out. However, the inefficient pushing or forcing of energy that drains you evaporates, and you experience the inspired action you take in sublime ways.

APPLICATION

At the end of each day gaze upon the Sublime Time glyph and know that you've done enough. You've been enough. Everything has had its now-moment in that day. All your projects are multi-dimensionally connected. They continue to evolve by you being deeply fulfilled and satisfied with your day and by just being. Focusing on the eight thousand items on your to-do list that didn't get done perpetuates the perceived lack of time. Instead, choose to honor yourself by acknowledging your forward momentum and appreciating what unfolded during that particular day. Declare that your time is sublime.

Another way you can apply this code is to pay yourself first with time. Set your priorities, with the must-dos—or what we like to call "to-joys"—on top. If spending time with your family is what matters most to you then that's a non-negotiable. You make spending Sublime Time with your family a top priority. If exercising deeply nourishes you, don't slot that in with whatever time seems to be left over from other activities. Make moving your body a priority as a creator being. Be very present in all that you're being and doing to cultivate even more now-moments of Sublime Time.

3
Divine Relationships

"All relationships are Divine."

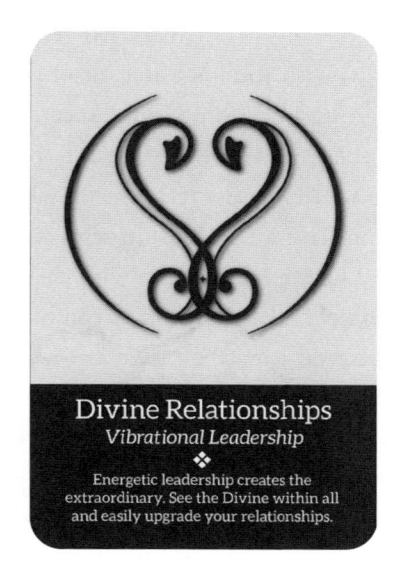

Divine Relationships
Vibrational Leadership

Energetic leadership creates the extraordinary. See the Divine within all and easily upgrade your relationships.

When we use the word *Divine,* we are referring both to Source, God, Goddess, Great Spirit, All That There Is, and also divine as in extraordinary. Your Divine Relationships are multi-dimensional, simultaneously extraordinary and Source-infused. Relationships are a resource of abundance that touches your entire lifetime and a source of great joy.

This code recognizes that you have different spheres of

relationships—with yourself, Source, and others; personal relationships with friends, family, animals, the Earth, and community. You may also enjoy professional or business relationships with clients and coworkers, as well as delight in your spiritual relationships with Source, guides, and your own self as a love being. Within each sphere of relationships there are varying degrees of proximity. Some are very close wherein you play a primary role in one another's evolution, and others are more on the periphery and everything in-between. All relationships have a purpose and may be with you for a lifetime or a season.

One of the greatest forms of abundance that is awakened with this Magdalene Code is the relationship that you have with your manifestations. You have a relationship with the book that you're writing. You have a relationship with your business as a being of light. You have a relationship with that which seems to be an inanimate object, like your home. You have a relationship with your finances and time. You have a relationship with the city you live in and with the Earth. This extends to animals, nature, and food. There are a multitude of relationships that you have on the physical plane.

You also have energetic relationships with the Magdalenes, beings of light, guides, Source, universal principles, and states of being. You have a relationship with your mood, body, and energy. You have a relationship with the resource codes of Yummy Money, Sublime Time, Divine Relationships, Radiant Energy, and the Magdalene Codes of Love.

Relationships are everywhere. Cultivating Divine Relationships is an incredible resource because whatever you're choosing to manifest won't bypass relationships. It will come in some way to a form of relationship. Relationships have the potential to accelerate timelines on the physical plane. Let's say you have a project the focus of which is to make a difference in the lives of a hundred people this year in a really deep and meaningful way, and you only have twenty-four hours in the day like everyone else. However, you can multiply your results and what is possible in twenty-four hours by having the support of other individuals, by cocreating, by partnering, which is essential to the new paradigm and which will assist you in your mission.

Your mission is unique to you. The relationships that you require will be unique to you. You may require primary relationships with light beings, animals, nature, and crystals. Recognize that your mission, just as it requires money, time, and energy, also requires relationships. The Magdalene Codes invite you to open your heart, get out of the "do it alone" mentality, and be in extraordinary relationships.

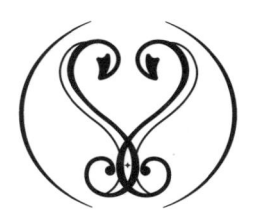

DIVINE RELATIONSHIPS RESOURCE
Vibrational Leadership

❖

Energetic leadership creates the extraordinary. See the Divine within all and easily upgrade your relationships.

The Divine Relationships Code is a fierce call to curate and actualize extraordinary relationships of true partnership based on Source energy. This code encourages you to circulate more divine energy in your relationships; to see the Divine in your creations, in yourself, and also in someone you may have friction with. Allow and amplify Source energy to flow in all of your interactions, those that are seen and those in the nonphysical realm.

As more Source energy flows into your relationship with yourself, you reclaim your innate capacity to be a vibrational leader; to lead and model from multidimensional energy. Vibrational leadership is where you focus your vibration in the direction of your true north, your heart and soul's knowing, and your deepest desires. This code assists you in leading yourself in the creation of that which you truly desire. As you focus your energy, attention, and action toward what you desire, the universe and those around you respond in kind.

When this card comes into your spread it may be an indication that you have deferred your leadership to an outside source and it is time to take back the reins of being a creator who is fully grounded in your seat as a vibrational leader. It may be that you have underestimated the potency of your presence and the ripple effect this has had and continues to have, not only in your life, but also in those around you and the larger evolution in consciousness. Vibrational leadership is where you are a leader who honors all around you and you model what is possible through the multidimensional field of love that surrounds you and your projects.

APPLICATION

When you are connected to Source every day you're in a high vibration, which magnifies your results on the physical plane. Plus, it feels divine to be aligned with the Divine, within and without. You may feel called to create a Divine Relationship spread to deepen your Source Union, or to amplify your connection with the Magdalenes, your manifestation team, and your higher self. As a Magdalene it is innate for you to have primary and vital relationships with the multidimensional planes and love beings.

Perhaps you would like to have a deeper connection with your guides, or you have a question you would like to receive direct guidance on from your higher self or the Magdalenes. Cultivate your question and draw as many cards as you are called to. Then spend a few minutes gazing at the glyphs before closing your eyes, gently relaxing. Notice your sensations and see what arises. The guidance may come right away, in a dream, or through an experience the next day. Be sure to write down the impressions, guidance, and clarity you receive.

4
Radiant Energy

"All energy is radiant."

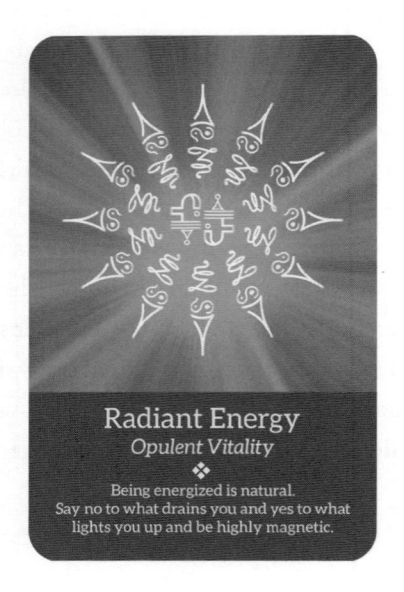

Radiant Energy
Opulent Vitality

Being energized is natural.
Say no to what drains you and yes to what
lights you up and be highly magnetic.

As you continue to explore the four primary resource codes, you may realize that one in particular seems to have been a thorn in your side. This resource may have been in a state of lack or eluded you in some way. Maybe, before working with this Magdalene manifestation deck, you've had an absence of energy. You've had low energy. There has been a fear of not having enough energy, vitality, or life force to get through the day, or to fully realize your project. This may have been your go-to repetitive pattern in the old paradigm and it has had a higher purpose. You can send love and appreciation to any moment that you experienced a lack of energy, time, relationships, or money, and be willing to have a new set point; to create a new relationship with this resource.

Radiant Energy is your birthright. Energy is infinite. Time is infinite. Money is infinite. Relationships are infinite. The source of energy is infinite. In survival lack-based consciousness you have been conditioned to think that your energy is like a jar of energy and you spend it like a battery. With this line of thinking, when you do something, energy is taken from you, for you have only a limited jar of energy to begin with. In this mode of operating you are in a constant state of managing and watching your energy to see if your battery is low.

This relationship to energy is based on a false premise. When you're tapped into the infinite supply of Radiant Energy, which this code supports you in doing, you're accessing a wider eternal divine Source of energy that is fueling all that you do.

We're not encouraging you to override, overextend, or push through—actually quite the opposite. Most likely as a highly ambitious lightworker you've come to this card deck from a place of depletion in your life. Maybe you've been pushing too hard, had low energy, or experienced burnout. We're not suggesting that you ignore taking care of your body and rest. Actually, we encourage the inverse—the Magdalene Codes are about replenishing, resting, rejuvenating, and emanating your natural radiance. Part of that is unhooking from the illusion lie that you are like a cell phone battery: as long as you're moving the battery is emptying.

Instead, you're invited to tap into this ongoing self-resourced, recharging-in-the-now-moment kind of experience.

Radiant Energy is a resource that is directly tied to the success of your manifestations and also your experience of the journey. We've chosen Radiant Energy because it has less of a charge than "health." For example, we could have said Radiant Health, yet health is not as expansive as energy. We're talking about your vitality, life force, enthusiasm, passion, and energy—your signature energy, for you *are* energy.

Your Radiant Energy fuels your health, absolutely. Your Radiant Energy is one of the supersecret keys to being a manifestation master. When Radiant Energy is running in your system you're highly visible and magnetic. When Radiant Energy is running in your projects, your projects take off. Whether you've experienced having a ton of energy in this lifetime or this is one of your areas needing attention, or anywhere in between, know that this Magdalene being supports you in becoming a being of Radiant Energy.

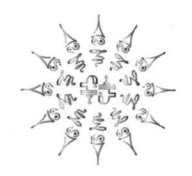

RADIANT ENERGY RESOURCE
Opulent Vitality

❖

> Being energized is natural. Say no to what drains you and yes to what lights you up and be highly magnetic.

Radiant Energy is enhanced by all the codes and vice versa. Experiencing Yummy Money, Sublime Time, and Divine Relationships enhances your Radiant Energy. Experiencing Vibrational Visibility supercharges your Radiant Energy. Star Love supercharges your Radiant Energy. Embodied Radiance supercharges your Radiant Energy, as does Ecstatic Bliss.

All the Magdalene Codes are nourishing to your Radiant Energy, and they imbue your creations with Radiant Energy. Your Radiant Energy is a given. It's a birthright. You can think of the resource codes and love codes as a birthright. When you draw this resource code of Radiant Energy it's a reminder that your energy is already whole, perfect, and complete. To actualize Radiant Energy you can simply come back to your birthright, using a gentle discipline. It doesn't matter why you left or what got you out of it. This is analogous to potty training a puppy and the puppy goes off the paper you have given it to pee on. All you do is bring the puppy back to the paper. Just bring yourself back to the "is-ness" of Radiant Energy—for again, it already exists.

The second message is that your system is directing you toward radiance all the time. Your life is directing you to radiance all the time. The love technology of the Magdalene Codes is deeply associated with Magdalene beings of love such as Anna, grandmother of Yeshua. You can think of these codes as energetic elixirs that create vitality within you, as well as the return, resurrection, rejuvenation, and regeneration of Radiant Energy.

This card steps forward to call you to recalibrate your energy signature in order that you make more efficient and expansive uses of your energy. It asks you to open up the receptor sites of giving, receiving, and having so that all that you do is amplified with ever-growing energy. As you gaze upon the Radiant Energy glyph, it unlocks what you and your Love Conceptions know about Radiant Energy. This can create a reversal of deterioration and seal energy leaks that you may or may not be aware of.

APPLICATION

When this card comes into your spread you're invited to say no to what drains you and yes to what lights you up. First, become clear on what is draining you by writing it down. Remember to include both internal thoughts, feelings, and old-paradigm ways of operating, as well as external activities, habits, and relationships, for instance. Go over your list and see if you can eliminate, delegate, complete, or shift the inefficient uses of your energy.

Then write down what lights you up, both internally and externally. Go over that list and see how you can add more of these activities, relationships, thoughts, and behaviors into your life. When you focus on what you're adding rather than what you're subtracting, the slower vibrational activities and ways of being have a tendency to go into a different dimension, one in which you no longer reside.

Twenty Codes of Love

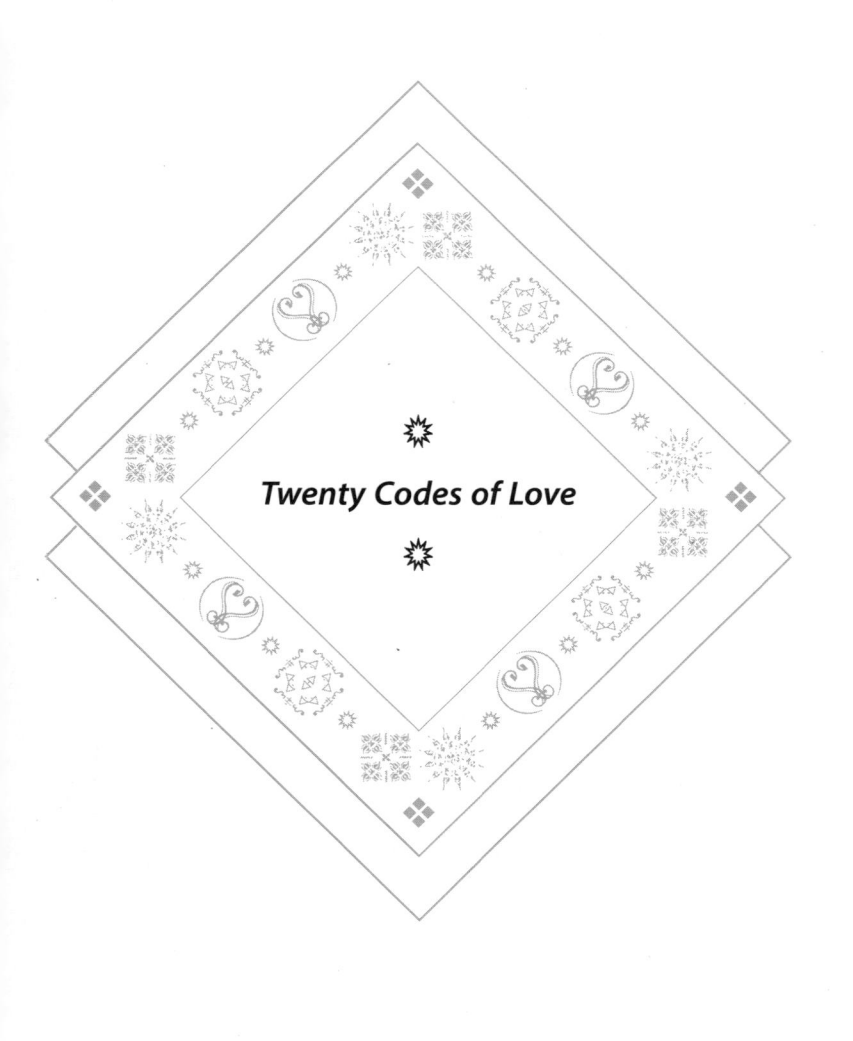

5
Love Conception

"I am conceived from the inner sanctuary of Source."

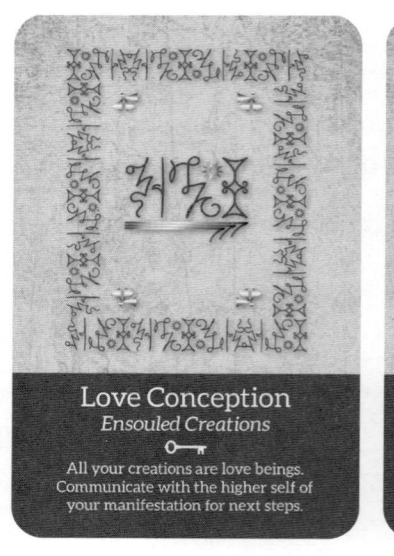

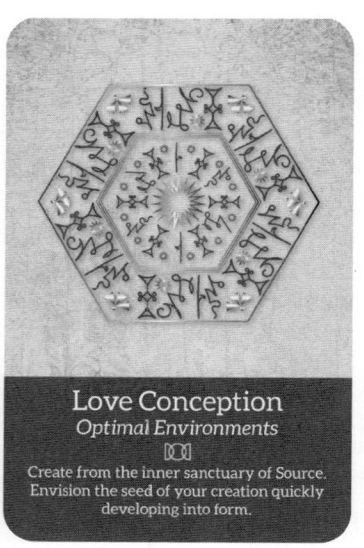

Love Conception
Ensouled Creations
All your creations are love beings. Communicate with the higher self of your manifestation for next steps.

Love Conception
Optimal Environments
Create from the inner sanctuary of Source. Envision the seed of your creation quickly developing into form.

All your manifestations created from Source are Love Conceptions. They are love beings—alive, dynamic, organic, and ever-expanding. This code reminds you to create from the primordial waters of Source as Source; to midwife your conceptions from the nonphysical into the physical with the full energy of Source intact. This way your creations are ensouled with infinite intelligence, a dedicated mission, and an abundance of resources.

The Love Conception Code ensures that you will have an optimal environment for all your creations to have a womb space in which to be created. As well, this code features a high level of magic, which is a Magdalene love technology, one where you conceive conceptions and create abundance through love. By using this code, you tap into the universal languages of love as well as the creator codes, including those associated with the quantum field, colors, numbers, sacred geometry, energy, frequencies, sounds, shapes, light language, glyphs—all the ways that the Divine within you and the source of all your creations vibrationally communicate. The love technology that is creating Love Conceptions is based on the vibrational matching of coherent languages of love and light, which brings unseen quantum particles into actualized consciousness in the visible physical plane, with the full energy of love intact.

Love Conception assists you in coming from the heart, wholeness, and from the sacred union of feminine and masculine wherein the journey and the destination are all based in the harmonic, inclusive energy of love. Each card spread is a Love Conception. Your day is a Love Conception. Your Multi-D Abundance—wealth in multiple areas that matter to your unique mission on this planet—is a Love Conception.

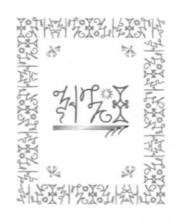

LOVE CONCEPTION KEY
Ensouled Creations

> All your creations are love beings. Communicate with the higher self of your manifestation for next steps.

Each of your desires is conceived in the inner sanctuary of Source. There are many beings of love present at this conception, whether you're conceiving a child or a business. Your creations are supported with everything required within and without to come into full fruition. The key glyph unlocks the spark or soul of the creation so it's manifested in wholeness.

All creations are formed from building blocks of creation or creator codes. Just as DNA is made up of the letters of ATCG, adenine (A), thymine (T), cytosine (C), and guanine (G), your Earth is created from the elements of Earth, Air, Water, Fire, and Akasha. Your manifestations are also made up of repeating elements. The ATCG repeats itself within the DNA, and depending on where it is read from it creates something unique, like an eyelash or a fingernail. All your manifestations are created from Source energy, which is a fractal repetition of different creator codes or languages of love (shapes, numbers, colors). This creates a physical emanation of what is essentially light, love, or energy. Anything you look at that is physicalized has a shape and a color, and may also be represented as a symbol or a number.

As you draw this card you are encouraged to tap into the fractal nature of being a creator love being, creating beings of love—your manifestations—with divine love, energy, and frequency. Speak directly with the infinite intelligence of your creation, higher self to higher self. Receive guidance as to the most aligned and efficient next steps required to bring your creation into form.

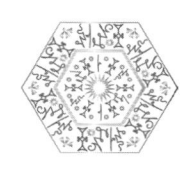

LOVE CONCEPTION HOLOGRAM
Optimal Environments

> Create from the inner sanctuary of Source. Envision the seed of your creation quickly developing into form.

The hologram glyph of Love Conception is a womb, a vortex of energy that you and your manifestations can steep within. The inner sanctuary is a very sacred place in a temple. It is, in essence, home to the most potent creative energies available. Creation requires a lush, fertile, conducive environment to come to full fruition. This code supports your system to rejuvenate, regenerate, and become an optimal environment that allows your manifestations to morph into form. It also provides a gateway in which the seed of your Love Conception can be fertilized with the Divine Masculine spark of the key glyph, and the egg or the hologram glyph, in a way that you are always hitting the bullseye of your target (your desired manifestation).

Love Conceptions, conceived in the inner sanctuary of Source, are spot-on. When you draw this card you are recalibrating to receive the optimal realization of your divine desires, beyond what you could even imagine. This may be an indication that it is time to fertilize your creations with loving thoughts and appreciation and surround yourself with uplifting individuals, weeding out negative self-talk or distractions that may be pulling on your energy. Pay special attention to cultivating a loving environment for your creations to come into form, which you are doing by creating energy vortexes using the card spreads.

Remember, you are not called to manifest something simply for the sake of having more. For the unquenchable thirst of separation consciousness says that there is never enough, that you are not whole, and the only way to be whole is to create more "stuff." This hologram reminds your entire system that this is an illusion lie. You *are* whole, you *are* divine, and you *are* choosing to engage in the act of creation as a creator being because it is natural for you to create. Create from love, align your journey with love, set your compass and the destination to the true north of love. Then all that you manifest will come from love, as love, to love in the most spectacular, conducive environment.

APPLICATION

Choose something that you would like to manifest on the physical plane. Go within your heart and call upon the masculine Magdalene Love Conception being and the feminine Magdalene Love Conception being and the inner sanctuary of

Source. Call upon the Magdalene love technology, which is the capacity to create Love Conceptions. Ask that the seed, egg, hologram, or blueprint of your manifestation comes into the womb of the inner sanctuary of Source. Ask that the activator, sperm, key, or spark of your manifestation comes into the womb of the inner sanctuary of Source. With as much love as you can muster, conceive the love being that is your creation, bringing together all the elements that it requires. The spark and the seed come together to conceive the embryo of your manifestation. It is fed, nourished, and developed with optimal nutrients and building blocks along the way. Your Love Conception is conceived with all that it requires and desires, magically calling to it the optimal individuals, circumstances, and resources that it requires to come into full fruition.

Notice if any part of your system is creating from a place of lack or settling for what you think you can manifest, which may be creating an unnecessary energy leak and ceiling on your Love Conception. If so, state this affirmation out loud: "I am conceived from the inner sanctuary of Source. This manifestation is a love being conceived in the inner sanctuary of Source." Feel the alchemical gold within the glyphs alchemizing any slower vibrations and absorbing them into love, elevating your Love Conception back to its original state of wholeness. Know that all that is required to bring this manifestation into form is on its way to you. Steep, communicate with the infinite intelligence of your creation, and act. You have the love technology of the Love Conception assisting you along the way. Remember to enter into each now-moment as a pathway to conceive even more love on the planet.

So it is and it is so.

6
Magdalene Molecule

"I am divinely designed for love."

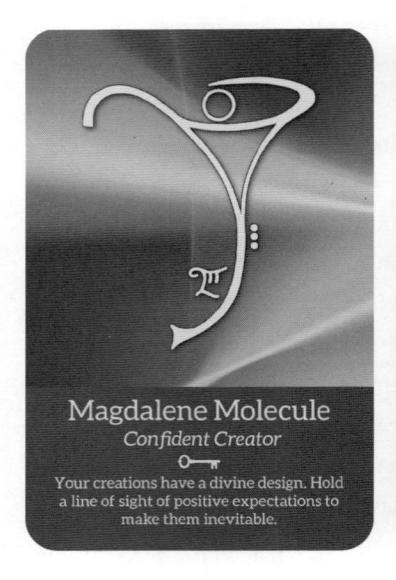

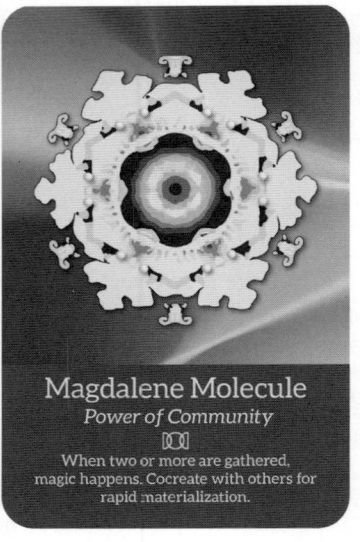

Magdalene Molecule
Confident Creator
Your creations have a divine design. Hold a line of sight of positive expectations to make them inevitable.

Magdalene Molecule
Power of Community
When two or more are gathered, magic happens. Cocreate with others for rapid materialization.

The Magdalene Molecule amplifies your connection to yourself as a Magdalene who carries a unique molecular structure that is designed for love. The love molecule makes you recognizable to other Magdalenes, magnetizing you to situations, individuals, and opportunities that will bring more love to all involved.

As you draw this Magdalene being in your manifestation altars, there is an invitation to tap into your inner radiance that glows like a crown of heart sovereignty. Your creations have a halo of love emanating from them, as do you. The Magdalene Molecule reminds you that love is natural, and you are designed for love. Within the coding of your DNA resides the molecular structures that are naturally coherent with the energy of love. This means that all that you connect with and create is enhanced by greater and greater states of love.

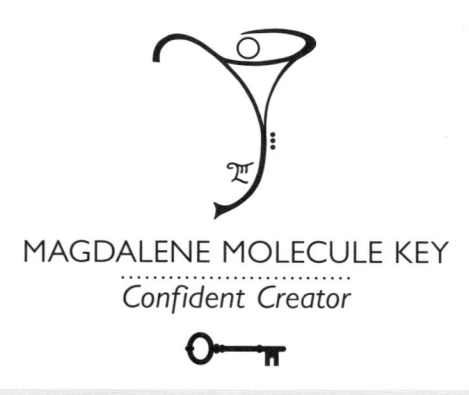

MAGDALENE MOLECULE KEY
Confident Creator

> Your creations have a divine design. Hold a line of sight of positive expectations to make them inevitable.

The Magdalene Molecule has a royal, confident, beautiful, radiant emanation. A crown or halo glows around your creative project, naturally magnetizing other molecules to gather, to come home, to be warmed by the hearth of love. Be confident that your creations will be realized and well-received. They have a higher purpose and divine design, as do you.

This card reminds you that the illusion lies of being worthy or unworthy, or enough or not enough, is not even a part of your energy field in unity consciousness. The unbalanced masculine energy may have shown up as a disavowing of the birthright of being supported and supportive. Maybe in the past you have played small, or not taken your full seat on the throne of your own royal sovereign lineage as a love being. Perhaps you have been hiding behind others or playing like a backup singer when you are actually a lead singer. The empowered masculine Magdalene Molecule key glyph reminds you that you are an advocate for love, that you are loved, and all your manifestations are an act of love. As such, they exponentially create more love.

Own your seat as a creator being with confidence and alignment without shrinking or having doubt in yourself or others. Be the lead in your own story; walk with the crown of your inner glow shining brightly. There is no one else like you and you are carrying a beautiful energy of high vibrational love for yourself and the planet. Be confident in your creations, for you are a creator being. Hold a line of sight of positive expectations to take your creations from a probability to an inevitability. You've got this!

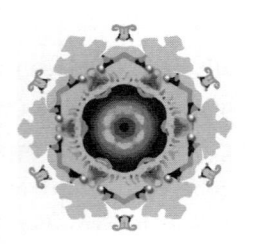

MAGDALENE MOLECULE HOLOGRAM
Power of Community

When two or more are gathered, magic happens. Cocreate with others for rapid materialization.

In order for your desires to manifest into physical form they must cross the threshold from energy into matter. A molecule is an electrically neutral group of two or more atoms bonded together. The feminine code as represented in the glyph is openhearted and reflects its open architecture. Note the deconstructed outer edge of the hologram. It's almost like a puzzle piece or a plug that has a perfectly matched shape, which can "dock" or come together with the absolute perfectly matched experience or synchronicity. Any manifestation is simply a result of this docking or coupling of energy.

Drawing this hologram code reminds you to move out of any "do it alone" mentality or a sense of being attached to an outcome. This may be a reminder to ask for help, to know that when two or more are gathered together, more becomes possible. Are you being called to delegate and exponentiate the speed at which your vision comes into form? Can you do this with support from others? Is it time to hire someone, call a friend, or expand your community? Remember, your creations are tied to a larger mission and most likely require energy, time, and the applied skills of others. This card is an indication to tap into the power of community to support your mission.

It's time to permanently shift what may be repelling support so you can be magnetic and, as such, bond deeply with others, and so that your creations are also magnetic and deeply bonded to the elements required to actualize. The old-paradigm illusion lies may have you unconsciously holding out support, thinking things like *It's easier to do things myself,* or *I can't trust others.* Thoughts like these, and a hesitation to ask for help when it's needed, often contribute to burnout.

When you draw this card take a breath and drop into your body. Has your system been running on a cocktail of stress hormones from too much suppressed feminine energy and unbalanced masculine energy? Are you unconsciously drawn to manifest your desire to feel the dopamine hit or adrenaline rush of cash or a recognition from others coming in? All of this is natural in the old paradigm. However, the new paradigm of manifesting honors the fact that it is your birthright to have all of your needs met, to be whole, to be nourished, and to have your mission in this lifetime be fully resourced.

The Magdalene Molecule has come into your manifestation practice to bring back the energy of neutrality, which is also the energy of love. You are divinely designed for love. The increase in units of consciousness of love in your system, a result of applying the Magdalene Molecule in your practice, creates an energetic magnet that naturally draws more molecules together so your creations can cross the threshold from energy into matter. This hologram, the Magdalene Molecule, invites you to have more community, support, and greater connection with others. You are a beacon of love. All will benefit from being in your presence, and vice versa. In this, you will be recognized as a Magdalene who carries the energy and lineage of divine love within. This code accelerates the materialization process by being a marker in the energetic template in order to draw in vibrational matches on the physical plane, thus bringing more molecules together to physicalize your manifestations.

APPLICATION

Your Magdalene Molecule in sacred union reminds you to radiate and emanate the energy of love. It asks you to know that you belong. You are a part of a larger council of ambassadors of love. Your mission requires abundance and reminds you to be neutral as this abundance comes to you. Let go of any idea of your abundance showing up in a certain way. Let this be reabsorbed into wholeness and be open to an even greater possibility.

Your money is a being of love that has a unique Magdalene Molecule that then draws more money to pool in your life. Your relationships carry the signature molecule of being a high level being of love that draws in more optimal relationships to pool in your life, which will in turn support your creation. As this card has come into your spread it is an invitation to have more support for your mission and your desires. The ways you're called to do this are unique to you. Perhaps you've created extraordinary results flying solo and you're guided to partner with a colleague you admire, or to train or certify others in your area of expertise. Maybe it is time to call in a new lover, friend, or pet, or to expand your family. Neutral bonding is based on the energies of win, win, win. The Magdalene Molecule assists you in coming together as whole beings with other whole beings. There is a shift from being stressed to being resplendently nourished and supported. The journey of your manifestations is flowing without any roadblocks because there isn't any judgment or lack that is driving the manifestation.

Use this code to accelerate your creations as they come into form, gathering more atoms into relationships so that the energy then unfolds and materializes in coherent ways.

7
Birthright of Love

"I am loved."

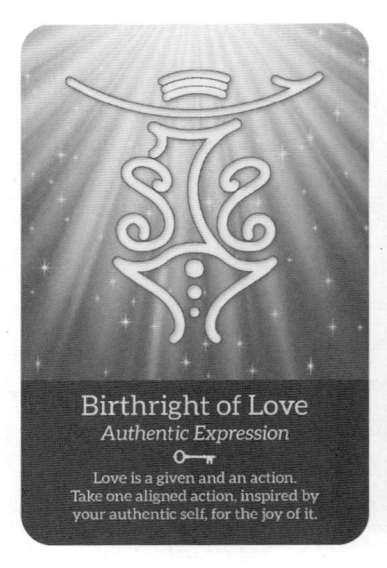

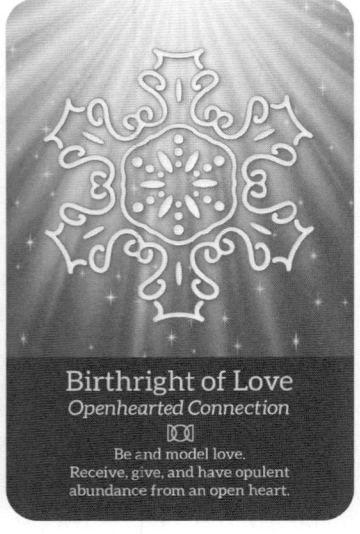

Birthright of Love
Authentic Expression
Love is a given and an action.
Take one aligned action, inspired by
your authentic self, for the joy of it.

Birthright of Love
Openhearted Connection
Be and model love.
Receive, give, and have opulent
abundance from an open heart.

The Birthright of Love is essential to new-paradigm living and manifesting, for the origin of all manifestations occurs from a solid knowing that you are loved. This instantly evaporates overlays that you may have unconsciously placed on your manifestations to fulfill something that is missing, or to prove that you are loveable. Love is a birthright; it is a given. As such, love is not something you "get" when you create success. Love is already there. It is not outside of you or something you have to twist yourself into a pretzel to receive. Love exists, and it is not contingent on having or not having money, impact, a myriad of relationships, good health, or however you may hold out love from yourself. Love is a given.

The Birthright of Love restores this idea first and foremost in your relationship with yourself, and it applies to all beings. You are loved, and so is everyone else. This code shines the light on the illusion lie that love resides outside of you, or within whatever you are choosing to manifest. It restores the universal truth that you are a creator being, with all that you require within. You are self-resourcing from an ever-unfolding, infinite supply of love.

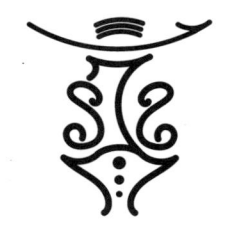

BIRTHRIGHT OF LOVE KEY
Authentic Expression

> Love is a given and an action. Take one aligned action, inspired by your authentic self, for the joy of it.

The masculine Birthright of Love Magdalene has an important message, which is that love is a given and it also loves to move. Love is an *act*. It is an action. It is a way of moving in the world that deeply honors self and others. This code adds an essential ingredient to your creative endeavors: choosing to create Multi-D Abundance is an act of self-love. It is a choice and decision to be in alignment with the natural birthright of the Divine, which is abundance.

If you haven't been manifesting your targets, most likely the root cause is connected to the Birthright of Love. All the codes are creator energies and are important; however, without the Birthright of Love in place, things will go a lot slower, and most likely be filled with friction. When you have the Birthright of Love in your energy vortex, imbuing your Yummy Money, Sublime Time, Divine Relationships, and Radiant Energy, there is a compounding effect that grows all areas of abundance in alignment with your free will and conscious choice.

You shift from unconscious patterns of trying to prove yourself as loveable or worthy. You shift from a state of believing that when you have X-amount of money or Y-amount of success you are loved, to a state of infinite self-love. This eliminates the illusion that love resides outside of you. Your actions, choices, purpose, mission, relationships, finances, health, body, home, and community are authentic and not based on earning love, because love is a birthright. This shifts patterns of approval-seeking, being guarded or hard on yourself, harboring insecurities, overcompensating, and perfectionism into ways of being that are self-loving and Source-resourced.

When this code comes into your spread and you lead your day from the Birthright of Love, you are secure and whole, respecting yourself and others. As a leader in the evolution of consciousness, you model what is possible. Perhaps you are a healer, coach, author, expert in your field, or a parent. When you connect with other individuals, who may be coworkers, clients, or family members, without having to prove anything to them or puff yourself up into seeming like a bigger, better version of yourself, they also have permission to show up as their authentic selves. When you are loved you take yourself and everyone else off the hook of filling some black hole of conditional love. "I am loved" is the affirmation associated with the Birthright of Love.

Your business thrives, clients get amazing results, and optimal experiences abound in your personal and professional life. The Birthright of Love is the secret sauce of opulent abundance without insecurities, projections, perfectionism, micromanaging, or hypervigilance running the show. Take one loving action today, not because you have to, but because it is natural for love to move *through* you. It is natural for the Birthright of Love to create momentum in the direction of your dreams.

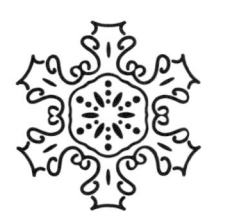

BIRTHRIGHT OF LOVE HOLOGRAM
Openhearted Connection

> Be and model love. Receive, give, and have opulent abundance from an open heart.

Love knows no bounds. Love is inclusive and expansive. The Birthright of Love opens your heart and nourishes your horizontal energy body, which widens your reach and impact in the world. In the old paradigm you may have put up walls, withheld love, or not received love. These protective mechanisms pinch off your connection with others and the natural circulation of opulently giving, having, and receiving infinite love and resources.

Many highly sensitive empaths shut down what's possible out of a false belief that when you manifest opulently you are not safe. Or when abundance comes to you, it comes with an overlay of fear, doubt, lack, or obligation, as a sort of indebtedness. Being openhearted supercharges your energy field, with the result being that slower vibrations don't enter your field. Being open, relaxed, and in a coherent state of being catalyzes the best possible outcome for all involved.

When the Birthright of Love joins your Magdalene Council, your project or creative endeavor is asking you to embrace even more the is-ness that you are loved, and that your creations are loved. Infuse the Birthright of Love into your creations.

Let's say you are a coach and you are writing a book. Without the Birthright of Love, you may have been bracing for a negative response to your work or you've been tamping down your desire and expectations that the book will be received with unbridled enthusiasm. There may be a lingering feeling of "imposter syndrome," or when it comes to spreading the word about your book you may pull back how many emails your send or posts you make, fearing that you may be an imposition or that there is something wrong with you. This is left over from the old paradigm and may cause you to hold back or play small.

The Birthright of Love restores vibrational wholeness to all relationships you are engaged in. When you meet someone new, rather than bracing for the likelihood that something could possibly go wrong, you know that you are vibrating at such a high speed that whether that individual likes you or doesn't like you doesn't even enter into your vibration. Love is not at stake in your negotiations and it's not at stake in the manifesting of physical plane resources. This is completely out of the equation, leaving you to be the most authentic you possible. You are not trying to force an outcome or talk someone into something, because you wouldn't dare—and it isn't possible anyhow.

You and your manifestations are loved. There is a certainty to this. As such, you can tune into the positive expectation that your mission is met with love because it originates in love and deeply connect with others from an open heart.

APPLICATION

Call upon the Birthright of Love Code at new beginnings: the start of a new project, the creation of a manifestation altar, or in the morning before your feet hit the floor. State out loud or in your mind's eye, "I am loved. All my creations are loved. Love is a given in this situation."

Imagine how your day would change if you simply knew that the energy of love was running fully throughout every moment of every experience you have. In this, love begets love. Abundance is a given and love is a given and the Birthright of Love naturally hangs out with the birthright of abundance. Love is multidimensional, having many expressions, facets, creative actions, and states of being. Abundance is multidimensional, having many forms. Abundance moves at a high vibration; love moves at a high vibration. They naturally blend together because they're in vibrational proximity to one another.

All that you desire is moving at a higher vibration. Radiant health, financial freedom, loving relationships, the fulfillment of your mission, being connected to Source and loved ones, and having an abundance of time to spend your way are all moving at a higher vibration. The Birthright of Love creates an environment wherein abundance and love merge because you and your creations are awash in a higher vibration.

8
Ecstatic Bliss

"It is a joy to be me."

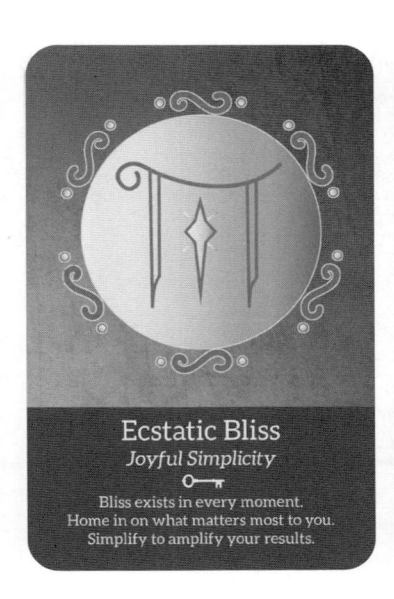

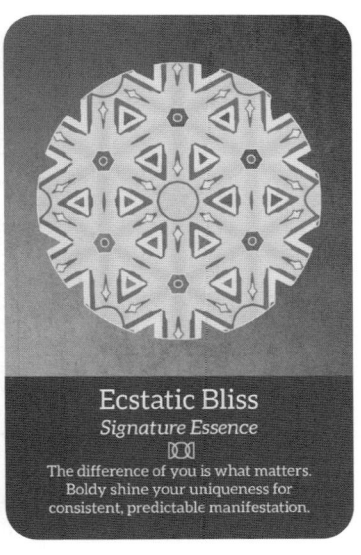

Ecstatic Bliss
Joyful Simplicity
Bliss exists in every moment.
Home in on what matters most to you.
Simplify to amplify your results.

Ecstatic Bliss
Signature Essence
The difference of you is what matters.
Boldy shine your uniqueness for
consistent, predictable manifestation.

The Ecstatic Bliss Code reminds you that bliss exists in each and every moment. It busts the illusion lie that pleasure and ecstasy are only connected to peak experiences, meeting goals, reaching targets, milestones, and celebrations, or that bliss is the effect of a cause. You do not need your desires to actualize to experience a pleasurable life; you can feel joy now. Bliss is autonomous and independent of what you do or don't do, eat or don't eat, create or don't create. The universal truth is that every moment houses the energy of joy, bliss, and ecstasy.

As you connect with this card you're invited to lighten up, to play, dance, sing, hum, explore, and not put off your delight until a later date like the weekend or retirement. Your entire physical experience is naturally designed to be enjoyed. The Ecstatic Bliss Code is a guideline to create from a place of pleasure and joy, not obligation and stress. It allows you to shift from excess or scarcity, too much or not enough, addictions and hit-or-miss joy to ever-present bliss that is unique to you and your mission.

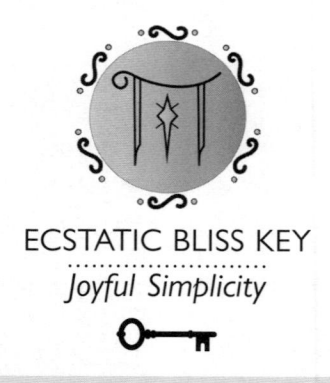

ECSTATIC BLISS KEY
Joyful Simplicity

> Bliss exists in every moment. Home in on what matters most to you. Simplify to amplify your results.

The masculine Ecstatic Bliss Magdalene reminds you of the simplicity of pleasure, the essentialism of joy. This key asks you to streamline and slough off that which is creating a complicated signal in your energy field. Return to the essence of you. Wealth is often elegant, simple, and straightforward. You may have been complicating your life by mingling your unique sweet spot of harmony with that which you have been told will bring you joy or is supposed to be blissful.

Perhaps in this lifetime it is not your choice or path to have a child, be in a romantic relationship, have family or oodles of friends, own a home, or any of the typical manifestations that you have been conditioned to think you need to be happy. Abundance is not a one-size-fits-all experience. You are the only one of you. What matters most to you and what you are aligned with will look, sound, feel, and radiate like you.

Being in a state of peace with the simple pleasures in life as well as the peak experiences and everything in between will assist you greatly. You may have abundance that no longer brings you joy or may feel like a burden. Perhaps you've outgrown it, or it isn't necessary any longer. This can be as simple as a favorite meal that used to bring you joy and now doesn't, or as complex as recognizing that your home is no longer in alignment with you. It is not about rushing to make external changes, although those will come if they're aligned and you choose to create them. It is about simplifying where you can. It's about essentializing. Essential oil is a very potent form of a flower. Focus on the essentials.

When this code comes into your day, it's an invitation to simplify to amplify your abundance. Go into your essence and take action to bring to completion anything that feels heavy or is weighing on you. Step out of activities, relationships, or forms of abundance that you've outgrown. There isn't anything wrong with the forms of abundance that are in your life, or the items that you own—it's simply that they may be tied to an older version of you. To be multidimensionally abundant is to return to your essence. It is to be current with who it is that you have become.

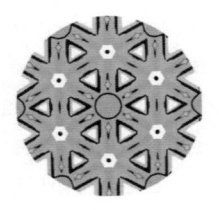

ECSTATIC BLISS HOLOGRAM
Signature Essence

> The difference of you is what matters. Boldly shine your uniqueness for consistent, predictable manifestation.

Bask, steep, dance, be, play, and breathe in the hologram of Ecstatic Bliss. Be in alignment with your unique, wacky, quirky, weird, pioneer self. Reclaim your inner rebel to guide you into bold moves that unleash your greatest joy. Bliss is not a prize. It is not an effect of manifesting; it is already in your life. The more you embrace bliss, the more you are in right relationship with the highest level of aligned abundance for you.

When you are in a dynamic state of joy, being your true self and dancing with life, you feel the most ecstatic. All moments are a dance. Manifesting is a dance of yin and yang, being and doing, play and action. Dance your signature move, sing your song, breathe your breath, and emanate your unique fragrance.

If you've drawn this card as a part of your manifestation altar you may have been pushing too hard. It may be a message to take a break, nap, rest, or simply *be*—to revel in the energy that is you without the expectation of needing to change.

Sometimes your system may interpret your desire to have,

be, and express more as a signal that there's something wrong with you. This is not the case. You are beauty, you are a kiss of divine bliss, you are the Venus rising within your core energy system. Your manifestations can't wait to be in your life! Make space for them. If your hands are full then you may not have the space you require.

Simple, elegant, streamlined. Steep in this hologram to reabsorb that which is no longer aligned with you so that it organically falls away, like leaves on a tree that know when it's time to fall with grace, ease, and an exhale.

What remains is Ecstatic Bliss.

APPLICATION

Go for a walk, get a massage, take a bath, rest, dance, sing, hum, hug, make love, eat, be, color, talk, enjoy, play.

9
Temple of Love

"I am a divine site of love."

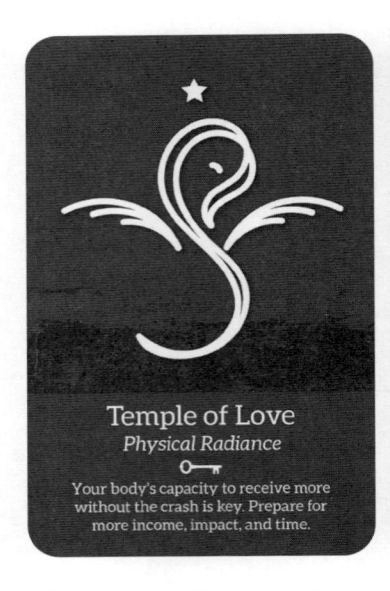

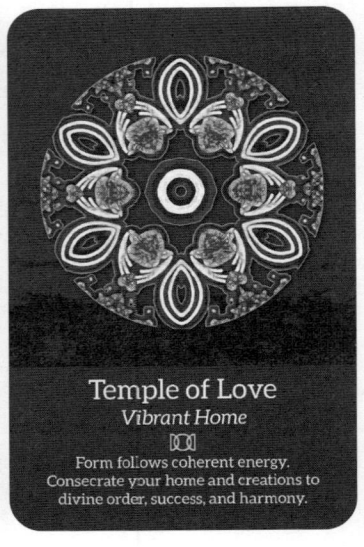

Temple of Love
Physical Radiance
Your body's capacity to receive more without the crash is key. Prepare for more income, impact, and time.

Temple of Love
Vibrant Home
Form follows coherent energy. Consecrate your home and creations to divine order, success, and harmony.

The Temple of Love Code encourages you to deepen into your sacred mission in this incarnation and connect to your galactic origin, your home star. Your resources in this lifetime are directly related to your divine mission that you carry across all lifetimes. When you draw this card you're encouraged to connect more deeply to your highest purpose in *this* lifetime. Infusing the signature energy of your home star into the divine blueprint of your mission and into your creations will multiply your results in the physical plane. Your Multi-D Abundance is directly correlated to this mission. The fulfillment of your purpose requires resources of time, money, relationships, and energy, and that which is unique to your experience in this incarnation.

The Temple of Love Magdalene holds a special place on your manifestation council, for there is a reconnection of "as above" (your origin star) with "as below" (your physical body). In the same way that the temples of Egypt are built as a reflection of the Milky Way, your experience on Earth is connected to you as a unique Temple of Love, and the origin star that is directly related to you and your mission. This alignment of home star with this incarnation's mission is depicted in the masculine glyph with the star above the crown. Claim and declare that you and your manifestations are sacred sites—divine sites of love.

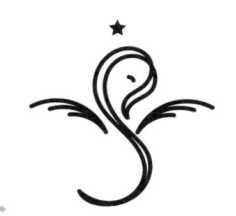

TEMPLE OF LOVE KEY
Physical Radiance

> Your body's capacity to receive more without the crash is key. Prepare for more income, impact, and time.

The masculine Temple of Love being is the key glyph that unlocks the blueprint of your divine mission in your DNA, the Akashic Records, and also in the higher planes. This connection to your home star automatically creates greater alignment and coherence in your system. When this card comes into your spreads you're encouraged to focus on your physical body to assist this process. Your body is asking to vibrate at a higher frequency on a regular basis. Your physical form is desiring an up-leveling that is coherent with the vibration of love. This may show up as a desire to move your body, drink more water, take salt baths, stretch, strengthen and tone your muscles, and support your nervous system to naturally hold higher states of abundance.

This way, as you create more abundance, your body is already operating at a very high level of vibration, and this incoming abundance has space to come into your life, into your body, without triggering a crash, burnout, or health issue. Your body is a temple and when it is a house of love you naturally receive more gracefully and frequently. When this card comes into your spread, contemplate how you can energetically and physically prepare for more. If you're creating more physical strength and your ideal weight, imagine the specific level of physical fitness and body weight that feels like a stretch and notice how your body feels. To facilitate this you may imagine yourself doing something that may feel impossible to your body (or at least your mind) like hiking the Camino or lifting your grandchild. Keep breathing and anchoring this in as a new norm so that when it does come in you will be energetically prepared. On the physical plane, this may mean hiring a personal trainer or being clear on what you will use the extra physical endurance for or tying it to your mission, knowing that your body is an instrument of higher consciousness. Anticipate your growth, and plan something nurturing to stabilize that growth. When you prepare for what's coming in, in advance, your expansion unfolds in delightful ways.

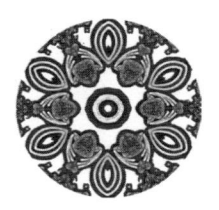

TEMPLE OF LOVE HOLOGRAM
Vibrant Home

> Form follows coherent energy. Consecrate your home and creations to divine order, success, and harmony.

The feminine Temple of Love being encourages you to take stock of your home environment. Your home environment is not only your physical body but also the temple that houses your physical body, the home that you live in. When this glyph comes into your spread it is an indication that your living space is asking for an upgrade. Specifically, it wants to be a harmonious, spacious, peaceful environment where the objects you have in it are current with who you are and your highest mission in this lifetime.

At first glance you may be drawn to declutter, spring clean, or move. This is the outward expression of the Temple of Love rippling into your home environment. The form of your possessions will naturally want to come into greater divine order. This may be akin to a magnet that brings iron filings that are in a chaotic pattern into a straight line. Creating more space in your home, closets, cabinets, and digital files opens up receptor sites in which your Love Conceptions may be birthed. As you go deeper into this code you are also called to upgrade the energetics of your home and your inner emotional state and heart coherence.

You may feel called to do a manifestation spread specifically for locking in a higher vibe in your mood and the energy in your home. Enjoy!

APPLICATION

You are a divine site of love, and your Love Conceptions are divine sites of love. They are Temples of Love. This code is a foundational member of your manifestation team and a high level of magic, for your creations are also Temples of Love. Each is consecrated with a unique purpose and higher mission.

When you are clear about what purpose you are consecrating your creations for and with, a fire is lit in the universe to bring you the supportive, cooperative components so that this is Fully Realized. Let's say one of your creation projects is to call in Sublime Time. When that Sublime Time Temple of Love is consecrated with a purpose it will come to you much more easily and quickly. Where is the time going to be spent, what is the purpose of it, are you going to spend more time with loved ones, doing things you love? If you had 20 percent more time to spend your way, what would you be doing, and who would you be spending it with? When you create a chamber in your Sublime Time Temple of Love that is specifically for a project like having more time to spend your way (hiking in the mountains, three-day weekends with your loved ones, or taking that transformational program you've had your eye on), the blueprint vibrates in a more coherent way and easily enables you to leverage time for these purposes.

In addition to consecrating your creations with purpose, connect your Love Conceptions with their origin star. All your creations emanate from Source and have a specific vibrational origin—what we also refer to as your home star. When you use your intention to align your body as a Temple of Love to your origin star, this accelerates the speed in which your creations come into form. This is compounded exponentially when you also connect the Temple of Love or sacred site of the being of light that is your creation to its home star. Even if you aren't consciously aware of what that may be, connecting your creation as a Temple of Love with its origin in the cosmos will create a divine order and facilitate change at a rapid pace.

This is the art of creating ensouled physicalizations by infusing higher plane energies into the physical plane, which is the heart and soul of this Magdalene manifestation system. To do this gaze upon the key Temple of Love glyph and imagine the star above the crown of the masculine Temple of Love representing the home star of your creation. Then visualize your creation crowning into the birth canal of the third dimension with a star above the crown. Then state out loud: "I choose to consecrate my Temple of Love creations with their higher purpose and connect them to their origin star for the highest and best good of all."

10
Infinite Love Meridian

"I am plugged into the infinite supply of love."

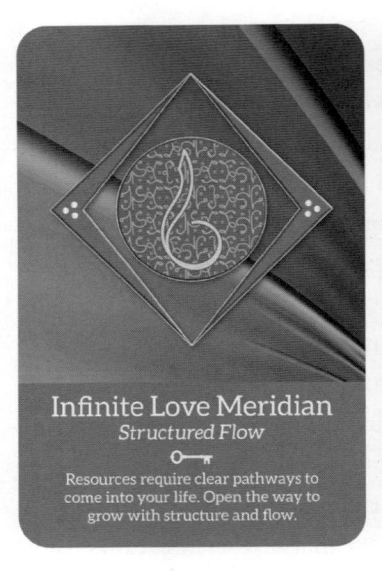

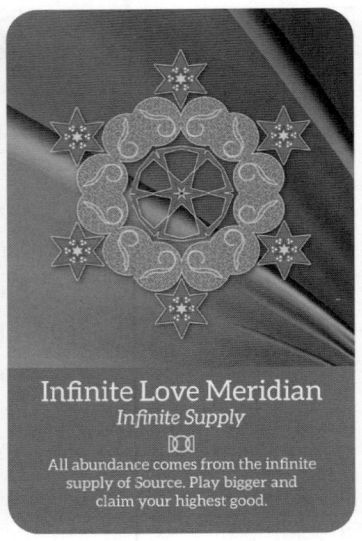

Infinite Love Meridian
Structured Flow

Resources require clear pathways to come into your life. Open the way to grow with structure and flow.

Infinite Love Meridian
Infinite Supply

All abundance comes from the infinite supply of Source. Play bigger and claim your highest good.

The Infinite Love Meridian taps you into the source of all your manifestations and shifts your focus from a finite amount of abundance coming from a limited source to one of being connected to the infinite source of all abundance, which is Source. A meridian is a pathway of energy that naturally flows through your system and the Earth, and illuminates the nonphysical network that connects All That There Is with all that there is. This network of meridians creates pathways between the physical and nonphysical. When you draw this card, it is an opportunity to amplify this magical network of connections to bring you into vibrational proximity with that which you are choosing to create.

Your manifestations are always much closer than you realize. At times they are simply looking for a pathway to find you, a meridian by which they may come into your life. This code is an invitation to expand. Perhaps it is time to create new streams of income, networks of relationships, a structure for your time, or ways for your energy and body to play. Open the way by taking action toward your dreams and being the individual who has what you desire.

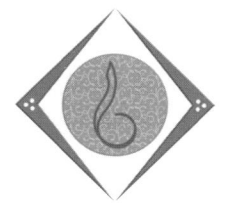

INFINITE LOVE MERIDIAN KEY
Structured Flow

> Resources require clear pathways to come into your life.
> Open the way to grow with structure and flow.

The key to creating expansion is simultaneously having wider pathways for resources to flow to you, as well as aligned containers to receive and nurture abundance so it stays in your life. Perhaps you've had a pattern of playing hot potato with abundance, where money comes in and goes right out again. Or supportive relationships enter your life and then quickly leave again. In order to sustain and expand multi-D wealth, it's important to widen your abundance muscle. Again, you can't channel an ocean of water through a small riverbank and store it in a thimble. Your manifestations are actualized from a combination of being connected to Source, having a pathway for good to flow into your life, and containers for it to pool within. The Infinite Love Meridian key code clears out energetic clutter, stuckness, and stagnancy, and aligns your system with structured flow so that you are tapped into an infinite supply of abundance that regenerates in your life.

Drawing this card constitutes an invitation to play an even bigger game, to expand your targets beyond what you believe is possible. If you've been playing small, hiding out, or pinching off your connection to Source and resources, you're encouraged to create bigger containers and playgrounds to play in. On the physical plane this may mean moving into a larger office space; opening a new bank account; creating additional streams of income, friends, exercise; or adding new activities.

If you've been too structured, micromanaging, overthinking, or overplanning you're guided to follow the energy, to get into states of superflow where you're led by your inner guidance. If you've been leaning heavily on being in the flow and avoiding having structures in place, your abundance is asking you to lean into the masculine Infinite Love Meridian to embrace the structures that will support all aspects of your creations. This way when money, relationships, time, purpose, and/or energy come into your life you are able to sustain this expansion and deepen into it. Combining aligned structure with inspired flow always out-creates manifesting with only structure or flow alone and ultimately leads to cultivating more abundance. Embrace the sacred union of the two.

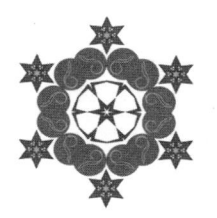

INFINITE LOVE MERIDIAN HOLOGRAM
Infinite Supply

> All abundance comes from the infinite supply of Source.
> Play bigger and claim your highest good.

This code reminds you to make internal shifts from approaching your manifestations and resources as finite to expanding them to be infinite. It encourages you to stop looking for your manifestations to come through specific ways but instead to open up to infinite ways of receiving. It is asking you to energetically connect your current resources (money, time, relationships, energy) to the infinite supply and source of these resources, which, as we've shared, is Source. Your current relationships, which have a set point of how much limited love flows between you, gets amplified with this code so that an infinite supply of love flows into those relationships. Your internal receptor sites begin broadcasting at a supersonic speed that is highly magnetic, calling your greater desires to you.

This code is an indication that you are ready to make a leap in your physical resources. In order to do so you are invited to tap into the infinite supply of love, and to open your manifestation meridians to be connected to all that you desire. You are asked to use the nonphysical energetic pathways and meridians as the shortest, fastest path to creating what you desire. For example, if you are choosing to dedicate your card spread and energy vortex to Divine Relationships and meeting a significant other, or finding a new team member or spiritual mentor, or creating a community of friends, on a soul level there already exists a meridian between you and those aligned individuals. A potential way for you to meet is by synchronicity or through your daily activities or referrals. This code and all the codes always honor free will and conscious choice of all involved so it is always a choice to meet and deepen relationships and also to end those that you've outgrown. And when you have this code running in your manifestation vortex, the energy of the Infinite Love Meridian is turned on so there is a surplus of love running in your system, in the nonphysical pathways that connect you to these optimal individuals.

You can come together in and from a place of wholeness. This upgrades your current relationships and also calls in soul-aligned perfect match ones, for there is no lack or fear in your vibration. There is a recognition of cocreation, of the sum being more than its parts, and an opening to the pathways that will accelerate your evolution and that of others. When you draw this card you are being asked to open your heart wider than you ever have before, to show up more fully, to play an even bigger game. You are being called upon to allow any past disappointments to be reabsorbed into the Infinite Love Meridian and to no longer be a reason why you limit what is possible. This code supports you in opening up the flow of infinite possibilities and magical energetic pathways to connect with the individuals, experiences, and abundance your divine mission requires.

APPLICATION

Write down or visualize your current resources: the money, relationships, work, and health you have. Not only the quantity, but also the quality of these resources. This is your current abundance set point. Now we invite you to connect the money being of love and your current money to the infinite supply of money and the source of money, which is Source. Connect your relationships to the infinite supply and source of relationships that is Source and go through all areas of abundance that really matter to you. Imagine and visualize that what connects your current abundance to the infinite supply of abundance is a meridian, a pathway, and that this meridian is widening to welcome in a higher quantity and/or quality of this resource. For it may be that you are currently satisfied with the number of people in your life and at the same time you'd like to deepen the connections you have with them. Ask that the unseen pathways that connect you with your manifestations is turned on more fully. This card, being in your energy vortex, creates a more direct and easier means by which you may come together and thrive as a result of the cross pollination of gifts, talents, and love you bring to one another.

11
Star Love

"I am fueled by my home star and the galaxies."

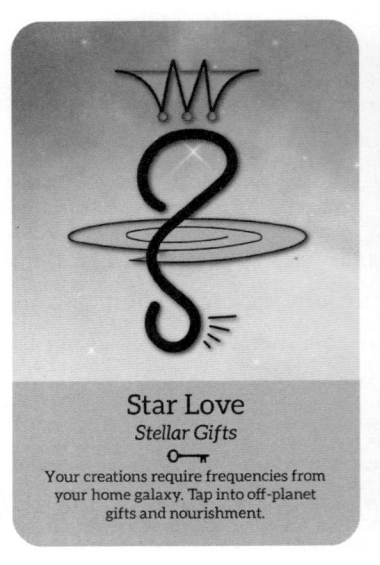

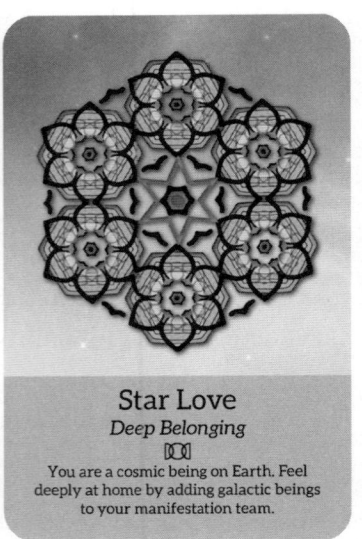

Star Love
Stellar Gifts
Your creations require frequencies from your home galaxy. Tap into off-planet gifts and nourishment.

Star Love
Deep Belonging
You are a cosmic being on Earth. Feel deeply at home by adding galactic beings to your manifestation team.

Star Love connects you to your home star so you feel at home on Earth because you're connected to your origin. You are a galactic being having an Earth lifetime. On Earth your system is nourished by water, air, food, relationships, exercise, sleep, love, learning, creating, meditation. Your galactic nature is nourished by frequencies and star consciousness that up until now haven't been accessible on the Earth Star. This may have led you to seek out substances that left you feeling empty or to have an unbalanced desire for more based on lack. With Star Love, this sense of being malnourished is now quenched with high vibrational frequencies from across the divine-verse.

This includes what we speak of as your home star, your origin, your source. Star Love reconnects you to these energies while you are currently in your Earth experience. This positively and radically shifts any sense of loneliness, of not belonging, or of feeling unfulfilled in your relationships or community. Instead you experience a deep sense of being at home, which emanates from understanding how to operate in the physical Earth plane while still being connected to higher dimensions. Star Love deepens your connection with guides, angels, and ascended masters.

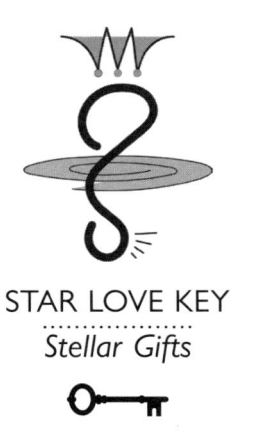

STAR LOVE KEY
Stellar Gifts

> Your creations require frequencies from your home galaxy. Tap into off-planet gifts and nourishment.

Remember, when you desire something it already exists in the energetic realms, the process of realizing this in the physical realm is one in which you vibrationally evolve to come into the same location as that which you desire. This code is especially useful when you have exhausted all angles and strategies to create something. Maybe you've had a health condition and no matter what you've tried it hasn't shifted. Or you've been "trying" to manifest a thriving career, loving home life, financial freedom, or vibrant energy and it always seems to be that the carrot is in front of you rather than in your mouth.

Your off-planet lifetimes are filled with adeptness, knowledge, and gifts you've carried during those lifetimes. Now that the Earth Star has increased her vibration, these galactic gifts can be used on Earth. These light technologies may include instant manifestation, telepathic communication, jumping timelines, creating through quantum entanglements, speaking your world into being, living on Earth as an embodied divine being, knowing how to uptake high quantities of knowledge and energy quickly, rapidly expanding and stabilizing it quickly, or being an ascended master of manifestation, healing, communication, or alignment. These gifts are unique to you.

When Star Love comes onto your altar it is time to stop trying to apply more effort, and get off the hustle train of do, do, do, and instead ask, What vibration is required for this to manifest? What off-planet knowledge do I have that I can now apply to this situation? What am I adept at that I can use in this situation to create what I desire? These types of questions are potent to ask before going to bed and you may choose to do a card spread before sleeping and ask to know the answer when you awaken. Ask to absorb the Star Love that your body, home, relationships, health, creativity, finances, play, and Multi-D Abundance require. The more you connect with Star

Love, the more deeply nourished you will feel. Creating from exhaustion, depletion, and striving are outdated ways to manifest. Star Love is like an energy spa for your soul.

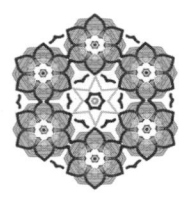

STAR LOVE HOLOGRAM
Deep Belonging

> You are a cosmic being on Earth. Feel deeply at home by adding galactic beings to your manifestation team.

On Earth you have been conditioned to think you are separate—separate from love, separate from connection, separate from others, separate from your desires, and separate from the Divine. Star Love is the antidote to separation consciousness, in particular when it comes to your sense of belonging and your innate birthright to exist and have what you desire. If you have been apologizing for your existence, feeling like you are an imposition on others, or isolating out of a fear of being kicked out of the community, losing love, being judged or rejected, then these slower vibrations are absolutely slowing down your creations.

It's essential that you feel at home in your own skin and on the Earth. As a lightworker, you know you come from the galaxies and are connected to many realms simultaneously. This may have created a sense of being so different that you've ostracized yourself from yourself. Star Love opens up the channels to your home star and galaxies so you are fueled with the energy sources that are natural to you as a spiritual and energetic being. This creates a deepened sense of the birthright to exist, to be a creator, and to have what you desire.

In addition to your relationships with others and yourself, you also have access to relationships with guides, light and love beings, ascended masters, planets, stars, overlighting devas, the Magdalenes, Source, and much more. Star Love opens up a deeper connection to your guidance, your council of Magdalenes, allowing you to actively partner with the aligned guides that are a part of your soul's journey and are also available to assist you in manifesting.

As you connect with us, beings of light and love in light and love, we are here to assist you in accessing infinite knowledge that is unique to you and your journey. We are delighted to commune with you and share inspiration that unlocks what you already know within you. When you draw Star Love, know that we are supporting your current manifestation project and that it is time to call upon an even more deepened state of nourishment and higher knowledge.

APPLICATION

Star Love is especially helpful when you feel tired, burnt out, or when what used to work is no longer working. It's also useful when you recognize that an unexpected or unorthodox approach is required. When you draw Star Love we invite you to connect to your home star, your origin. Ask that an energy vortex is created that will allow you to bask in the higher knowledge that you have in off-planet lifetimes and on other galaxies and star systems in alignment with your free will and conscious choice.

Notice that your path to manifesting may take you in an unusual direction, one that may seem circuitous. However, Star Love, your guides, and your higher self are opening up something that is even more effective than the tools you'd previously been using. This is a blessing and a very positive addition to your manifestation team. Enjoy the highly rich nutrients, a renewed sense of zest, and passion for your life. Also, consciously connect with your guides to assist you in all your endeavors.

12
Magic of Love

"I am a midwife of magic."

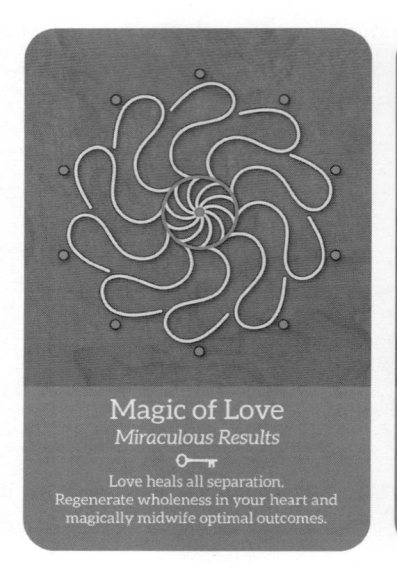

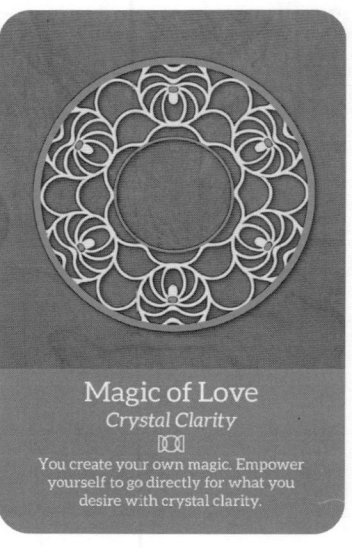

Magic of Love
Miraculous Results
○━┱

Love heals all separation. Regenerate wholeness in your heart and magically midwife optimal outcomes.

Magic of Love
Crystal Clarity

You create your own magic. Empower yourself to go directly for what you desire with crystal clarity.

Magic of Love addresses the original separation from Source, mends heartbreak, and lifts the separation consciousness stamp from the pain body. This code rejuvenates and restores the abundance body, physical radiance, emotional sovereignty, and repairs past and current life rifts in your field.

Magic and love have been a part of the bipedal's experience for eons. Where there is magic, love is present, where there is love, magic is present. This code is a reclamation of your magical prowess that emanates from love. It is an invocation to come into oneness with one of the most powerful energies available, divine love. When you love fully and as the divine being you are, anything becomes possible. Allow this code to restore and rejuvenate your faith in yourself, love, and in your creations. The movement that love creates is simply magical. Be enveloped within the sacred heart of Source and resurrect synergy and coherence in all dimensions where you reside.

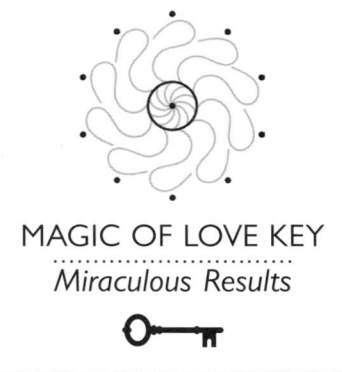

MAGIC OF LOVE KEY
Miraculous Results

> Love heals all separation. Regenerate wholeness in your heart and magically midwife optimal outcomes.

The Magic of Love Code is one that can transcend the heartache of a million lifetimes and it creates miraculous healing of rifts between families, coworkers, and within your soul. When this card joins your manifestation team you are in for a rapid shift for the better in your results. The Magic of Love is magical and creates an instant affinity between previously discordant energies. This means you can continue to create from a greater place of neutrality and surf above the emotional, mental, and physical ups and downs.

Magic is the essence of creation and manifestation, and

when you calibrate your desires with magical intent you create like wildfire. The key to the Magic of Love Code is to vibrationally move into the dimensions where your slower vibrational doubts do not reside. These codes are about movement—the movement that is naturally happening in your physical body to come into a state of homeostasis and heal itself. The movement and momentum your desires have are magnetizing and summoning to you the next natural steps in creating them. Get ready for the rapid and miraculous realization of your deepest desires.

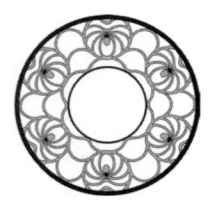

MAGIC OF LOVE HOLOGRAM
Crystal Clarity

> You create your own magic. Empower yourself to go directly for what you desire with crystal clarity.

The Magic of Love fractal hologram is an invitation to go straight for what you desire—to be clear in your intent and focus, and to align your energy and actions to that target. Crystal clarity is always within you. Drop into your inner knowing and identify the next steps, which may be to simply be or to act. You always know. The Magic of Love encourages you to stop waiting and start creating. To know and go.

Your projects are surrounded by love and magic. The Magic of Love hologram simply amplifies the environment around you and your projects so it becomes palpable to you that magic is afoot. Remember, you create your own magic; you are the creator of your results. This card is a reminder to take back your power as a creator if you have unconsciously deferred it to a source outside yourself.

Magdalenes have been known for rapid healing, longevity, youthing (reversing aging), high quality of lifespan, and life force energy. The Magic of Love hologram can also be a field of energy in which you rejuvenate, regenerate, and come into greater Radiant Energy. This is not only the case for your physical body but also for your relationships, projects, and internal state of being. Perhaps you have lost the passion in your career or marriage or you have gotten into a pattern of only going through the motions. The Magic of Love reignites your inner glow, and an outpouring of Radiant Energy is infused into all that you touch.

APPLICATION

As you gaze upon the Magic of Love glyph your core desire and passion for life is amplified. You're deeply connected to the source from which you came, and the higher purpose and mission for this incarnation. The Magic of Love reminds you of the steadfast truth that what you are up to (including realizing your creations in the physical plane by amplifying your magical capacities on the higher planes) is much vaster than you.

This is a good thing, for when you tie your desires to a

greater *why* then more becomes possible. When this card comes onto your manifestation altar take a few moments to connect to the desire underneath the desire you have. If you desire more money, why do you desire that money? Is it to have more freedom, to create an even bigger impact on the planet, or . . . ? What would you do with that money? Give it a home, give it a direction, map it out. If you desire more or better relationships, why is that? What is the deeper desire and reason why that matters to you? Is it because you have forgotten your Birthright of Love and are seeking this love outside yourself? Is it because you get to experience more facets of yourself and enjoy the facets of others when you are in relationship with them? When you connect to a deeper *why* you naturally uncouple from any resistance and start an inner fire that creates magical results.

Invite the Magic of Love to cascade magic and love into all that you do so not only do you realize what you desire, you also actualize the desire underneath the desire. This way your journey and destination are one.

13

Magdalene Heart

"I am a magnificent receiver."

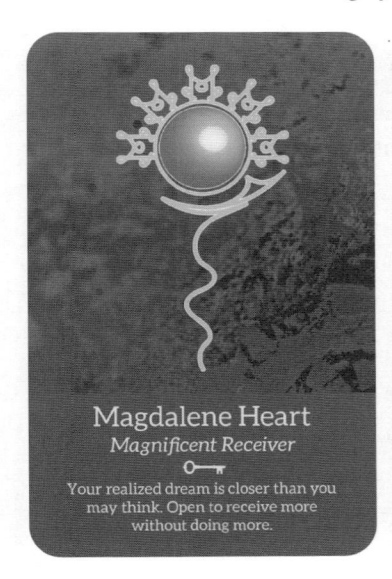

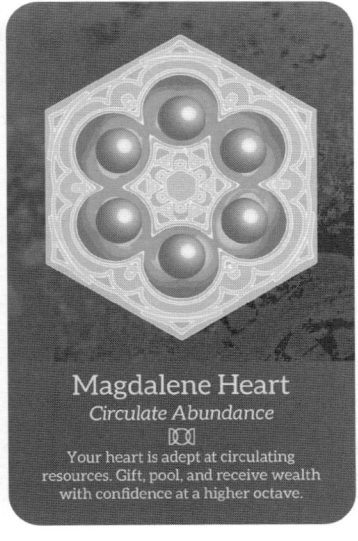

Magdalene Heart
Magnificent Receiver
Your realized dream is closer than you may think. Open to receive more without doing more.

Magdalene Heart
Circulate Abundance
Your heart is adept at circulating resources. Gift, pool, and receive wealth with confidence at a higher octave.

The Magdalene Heart opens your heart and horizontal field to be vessels in which to incarnate more of your vertical nature. When you bring the feminine and the masculine receptivity, the internal and external, the horizontal and vertical planes together, you are in the seat of the highest divine service. It is natural for you to ooze contribution, to be a fountain of inspiration, guidance, and a light for others. The Magdalene Heart provides a vessel for your higher consciousness to be in constant communion with your

Earth Star experience. It solidifies an unflappable connection to the heart of Source and your greatest divine service.

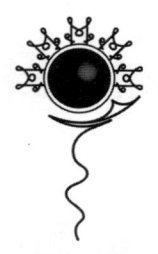

MAGDALENE HEART KEY
Magnificent Receiver

> Your realized dream is closer than you may think.
> Open to receive more without doing more.

You are innately a magnificent receiver. It is natural for you to receive. Receiving is as valuable as giving and having. All your creations must be received in order to come into fruition. You receive ideas, resources, guidance, and support all the time. Unlock the full breadth of your capacity to receive with this key glyph and notice what emerges.

There comes a point in your creation journey where your Love Conception is knocking on the door of the physical realm. Your dream is very close to being realized, all the actions have been taken, everything has been lined up, and the last step is to receive it.

The Magdalene Heart opens your heart, your horizontal field, and widens your receptivity a thousandfold. Opening the heart quiets the mind and eradicates interference, distraction, and reactivity, fortifying your system and your projects to receive even more all along the way. All that there is exists in each and every moment. Thus, your Fully Realized manifestation already exists in the now. It's time to open to receive that which is already there.

Perhaps this card is coming into your manifestation spread for Divine Relationships. You may have been receiving mediocre support from your team, coworkers, or family because unconsciously you were repelling rather than receiving. But being opulently supported with aligned partnerships already exists. Notice that when this card comes into your creations you will experience a shift from being disappointed in the support you receive from others to being pleasantly surprised at how the support you receive surpasses what you imagined was possible. The Magdalene Heart key code shifts your slow vibe or negative expectations so that you are calmly and confidently holding the best possible outcome in your field and in your heart. This calls out the best in others because it is a vibrational match on all levels of your system.

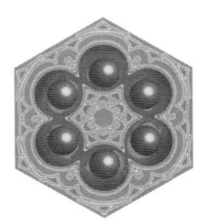

MAGDALENE HEART HOLOGRAM
Circulate Abundance

Your heart is adept at circulating resources. Gift, pool, and receive wealth with confidence at a higher octave.

The universe is always conspiring for your benefit and highest good. And it is always your conscious choice to receive and create your wildest dreams. The Magdalene Heart hologram creates a conducive environment for you to be wildly receptive and therefore wildly successful in what you place your attention on. The Magdalenes and these codes are based on maximizing the power of feminine receptivity and that of the energy realms. A lot can be materialized by simply receiving.

Being a magnificent receiver is also embellished with the energies of grace, gratitude, and delight. There is a childlike innocence to receiving as a creator being. Know that abundance is all that there is so when you receive you are actually in an infinity loop of receiving, having, and gifting simultaneously. In the new paradigm this is paramount to all your relationships and endeavors. It is a new way of being. Know that no matter what role it seems like you or others are playing you are all simultaneously receiving, having, and gifting. For example, you may be the coach that is leading a client so it seems like you are in the giving role, however, this is seeing "receiving" as being separate from wholeness. As the coach you are also growing from your client. It is not possible to give without receiving or receive without giving or have without giving or receiving, for the circulation of abundance is all interconnected. The Magdalene Heart restores this awareness.

This code supports you in confidently and consistently receiving more—more money, energy, love, creativity—plus to have and give more. If you've been feeling insecure about spending money on a project, receiving support from others, or allowing your resources to pool around you, this card is a nod from the universe to confidently take the next natural step that is before you.

APPLICATION

Place your hands on your heart and repeat the affirmation "I am a magnificent receiver" ten times upon awakening and before going to bed. Notice that this stance is a powerful, fierce, and loving way to be in the world. It's a code that you live by. The next time someone offers you a compliment, gift, or wants to pay for something for you, take a breath and say this mantra, and then say yes to the gift! Receiving is a gift.

14
Emerald Love

*"I am unique. I am true to myself.
I am a jewel."*

Emerald Love
Stabilized Expansion

Expansion is a given.
Quickly stabilize your growth so it is
natural for you to expand again.

Emerald Love
Bespoke Nourishment

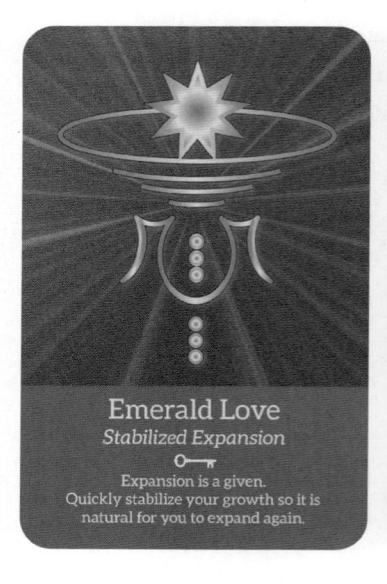

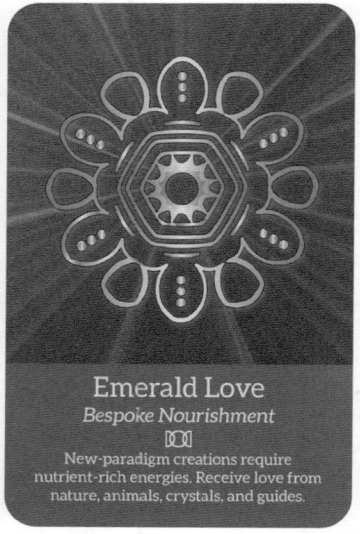

New-paradigm creations require
nutrient-rich energies. Receive love from
nature, animals, crystals, and guides.

Emerald Love amplifies your signature energy and stabilizes your higher dimensional self in form. This nutrient vibration relaxes your system and fuels all that you and your creations require as love beings. It naturally supports you in dropping less nourishing vibrations and habits because you are tapped into the core energy that is compatible with your Fully Realized self.

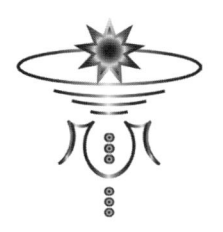

EMERALD LOVE KEY
Stabilized Expansion

> Expansion is a given. Quickly stabilize your growth so it is natural for you to expand again.

You and your Love Conceptions are unique energy in form, with a specific one-of-a-kind signature energy. Expansion, growth, and manifestation require nutrients. Emerald Love is superfood for you and your creations' signature energy to be emboldened, amplified, nourished, and glowing. When the unique signature energy of your creations as love beings glows brightly, all cooperative components rush in from across the multiverse, deeply nourishing your actualizations to continue to grow.

The Emerald Love card has joined your manifestation spread to call forth the energetic nutrients to stabilize and integrate your higher dimensional self—to restore your royal and divine line, your galactic divinity. This code acts as a cosmic eraser that brings into a place of completion anywhere there is inner conflict or a push-pull within you. For example, these two aspects may be your high-achieving masculine side and your receptive, being, feminine side, or your logical side and intuitive side. This code opens your vision to a greater field of awareness, bringing all the seemingly disparate parts of yourself into coherence, oneness, and synergy. This includes the fastest vibration of you, and your manifestations to the slowest vibration. By turning up the dimmer switch on your manifestations with this code, they are created with greater ease. This supports you in stabilizing your expansion, sustaining it, and then naturally expanding it again from a place of being deeply nourished.

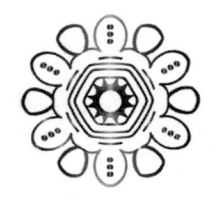

EMERALD LOVE HOLOGRAM
Bespoke Nourishment

> New-paradigm creations require nutrient-rich energies.
> Receive love from nature, animals, crystals, and guides.

Being in a state of coherence with yourself is hot, attractive, aligned. Rejecting yourself or berating yourself for being weird, wacky, different, and unique is the old-paradigm illusion lie of separating and divorcing from yourself. The difference of you is what matters (materializes). When you lean into what makes you different, unique, and out of this world, your difference makes all the difference to your bold actualizations, allowing them to come into form at an accelerated pace. This card invites you to color outside the lines, think outside the box, innovate and open to your intuition to illuminate the shortest, fastest path between what you've created on the higher planes and stabilizing and integrating (manifesting) it into your Earth experience.

The Emerald Love Code creates an energy vortex of "As above, so below, as within so without." It does this so that your love body is fueled by all facets of your being. This includes extraordinary nourishment from crystals, nature, animals, sacred geometry, colors, numbers, and light language. The key to unlocking this nutrient-rich boost to your manifestations is to embrace your uniqueness.

The guidance this card offers may seem anti-intuitive; however, listen to your deep inner knowing. Perhaps you are being guided to play with your pets, bask in nature, take a nap, massage your feet, or hold a crystal. These may not seem like needle movers when it comes to getting stuff done if you are looking at these activities from the lens of the old paradigm. However, recognize that in order for your creations to move forward you need to broadcast your unique signature energy and that of your Love Conception. The more the seed of your manifestation is nourished with energies bespoke, dedicated to and customized for you, the louder and clearer is the signal you broadcast. This makes it easy-peasy for abundance to come to you.

Authentic creation is what is being asked for at this time. Perhaps you have been trying to create in a way that actually drains you or isn't authentic to your true divine nature and essence as a soul. This code invites you to be radically honest with yourself, to deeply honor the jewel that you are, and to reclaim your unique way to create.

You may receive guidance that seems unusual, like cleaning

out a junk drawer rather than making a phone call that could lead to a sale. Or doing a puzzle, coloring, or blowing bubbles, which on the surface may seem unrelated to reaching your targets. However, enhancing your vibrational richness is essential to manifesting Multi-D Abundance. They go hand in hand; they are one. Allow this code to give an infusion of vitality to your projects and Love Conceptions and watch them grow before your eyes.

Emerald Love, including amplifying the difference of you, following your inner guidance, and exploring innovative ways to create, is a very effective and practical tool. What will nourish your creations today? What does your love body require and desire?

APPLICATION

Now is a time for you to innovate, pioneer, explore, play, and organize your now-moment from a coherent alignment with your multifaceted self. What is the most unique thing about you and about your desire? How does it seem to defy gravity or conventional wisdom? Amplify this difference and open to insights that take this difference even further into the realm of genius.

15
Orgasmic Creation

"I am in the joy of creation."

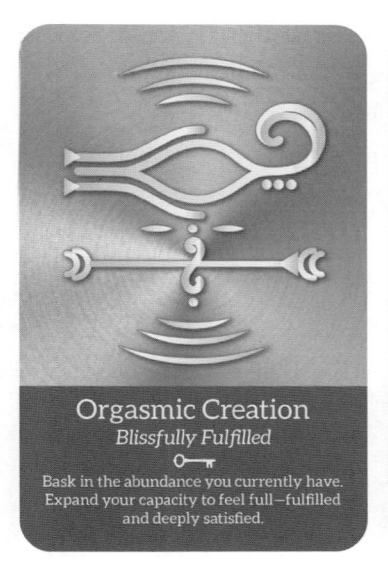

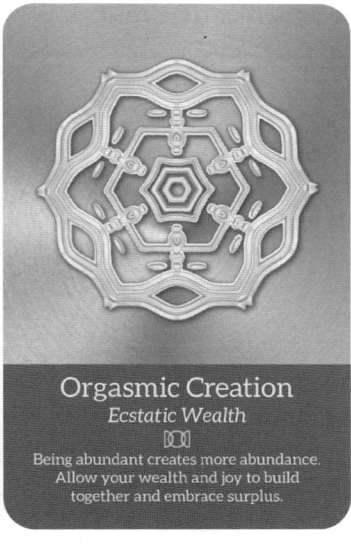

Orgasmic Creation
Blissfully Fulfilled
Bask in the abundance you currently have. Expand your capacity to feel full—fulfilled and deeply satisfied.

Orgasmic Creation
Ecstatic Wealth
Being abundant creates more abundance. Allow your wealth and joy to build together and embrace surplus.

Orgasmic Creation is a state of being, not something that comes and goes; it's creation as a given. Orgasmic Creation posits that you are in the inner sanctuary of Source as you create. You are one with the creative life force that animates all creations. Orgasmic Creation is generated from bliss in the now, rather than the illusion lies of hard work, trying to figure it out, or pushing. As an Orgasmic Creator, you are turned on, juicy, succulent, magnificent, fulfilled, and overflowing.

As such, your creation practice is not fueled by what gets created, although that is nourishing. Instead, your practice is fueled from the space of bountiful opulence of orgasmic, joyful creation. This restores your experiential capacity to be connected with Source and become whatever it is you have actualized. It means to be satiated and fulfilled by what you do create, including the experience of getting there, and to not be focused on the gap between where you are and where you're going. Bring your fragmented parts back together, allow this code to absorb any illusion of shame or unworthiness, and replace these with a palpable knowing that you can experience joy now, no matter what your external circumstances are.

You are bliss in form; you have been conceived on the physical plane of the masculine sperm and the feminine egg coming into sacred union. You have incarnated through the portal of sexuality and (at least) the male orgasm. On the higher planes the energy was also building into a climax of joy in response to your choice to incarnate. The details of your birth were impeccably chosen by you and those involved, with a perfect match to your parents, your soul's purpose, your gifts and talents, and the knowledge and resources you require to seed your heart's desires. Return the sacred union between your physical plane actions and rejoice in the higher planes of your Love Conceptions. Know that all you are creating also has a team of support on the energetic planes and on Earth.

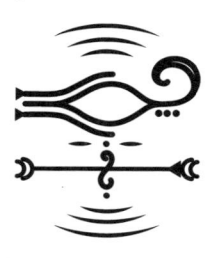

ORGASMIC CREATION KEY
Blissfully Fulfilled

> Bask in the abundance you currently have. Expand your capacity to feel full—fulfilled and deeply satisfied.

As a creator being continuously in the act and state of creating, there is a deeply satisfying, natural, and replenishing energy always building in your system. Creating is an optimal environment and an activity that is pleasurable, joyful, and ecstatic when deeply experienced. This card reminds you to slow down, in order to speed up. Remember to add in how the journey to your creations will feel. Let go of hard work and striving and ground into the impulse of creation. Creation knows how to create. You know how to create. Your creations know how to be birthed into the world; there is an innate intelligence and divine order to their creation.

Allow the energy of your creations to build and fold your internal state into your outcomes. For example, you are choosing to create x-amount of money, y-amount of relationships, z-amount of energy in ways that are delightful, joyous, and juicy to you. This infuses your creations with a high vibration of delight, joy, and juiciness that then exponentiates the opulent impulse of creation in ways that will positively surprise and satisfy you.

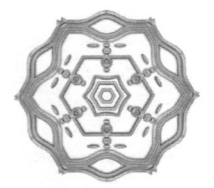

ORGASMIC CREATION HOLOGRAM
Ecstatic Wealth

> Being abundant creates more abundance. Allow your wealth and joy to build together and embrace surplus.

Orgasmic Creation is where your creations are infused with love and fueled by joy. This code invites you to make creating an art form or *practice,* like a yoga practice. You are already a manifestation master and an adept so it is not practice to get better at it, it is practice to explore, experience, and to allow the nectar of the Divine to bubble up into your awareness. Orgasmic Creation is taking an ecstatic breath to taste the essence of your creations. To build energy also means expanding your capacity to have.

Allowing pools of resources to build in your life, love body, and environment enhances your capacity to relish in growing abundance, to feel not only safe as your abundance grows but also delighted by the expansion. In the old paradigm, expansion may have been interpreted by your 3D system as being dangerous at times. If you have too much pleasure you may not be responsible or if things grow too fast you may find yourself alone at the top.

Regardless of what your monkey mind or safety patterning is telling you, when you pull this card you shift your focus from this unconscious creation to consciously creating from a place of fulfillment. Even if the sprouts of your creation seeds are not above ground where you can see them, rest assured something is always happening.

This is where you consciously bring your attention to the abundance you already have, to the surplus that's in your life. Let's say you are in the process of actualizing a sold-out event, bestselling book, or your first or next six figures, and you've sold ten tickets, or a hundred books, or brought in ten thousand dollars. Your brain will naturally have you focusing on the gap between where you are and where you want to be, which is the opposite of orgasmic.

Instead, practice being deeply fulfilled by the ten individuals who have signed up for your event, the one hundred readers you have, the ten thousand dollars that are in your bank account. Build your muscle of being satiated, fulfilled, and actually receive and integrate the good that's already in your life. Orgasmic Creation is a pattern interrupt code, one that calls out lack consciousness as an illusion lie and calls forth your natural state of being, which is joy. Ecstatic wealth comes from being deeply satisfied and fulfilled. When you operate from this stance, your life becomes very pleasing to you.

APPLICATION

Return joy, pleasure, and fulfillment to the exalted place in your heart's desire by having it be non-negotiable in all that you do. When you find yourself moving out of a satiated or blissful state (and you will), stop and restate the affirmation "I am in the joy of creation." Then guide your awareness into a practice of deeply appreciating the Multi-D Abundance you already have in your life. You can do this alone or with a loved one where you state out loud, "I deeply appreciate the loving relationship I have with myself, with you, with the guides. I appreciate the resources that are already in my life, the home I live in, the bed I sleep in, the money, energy, and health I currently have. I appreciate this appreciation practice. . . ." Just keep going until you notice a palpable shift within you into a state of grace and re-Sourcedness. The fastest way to permanently eliminate separation consciousness is to consciously and continuously be in a state of joy and fulfillment.

16
Magdalene Love Body

"I am vibrationally autonomous."

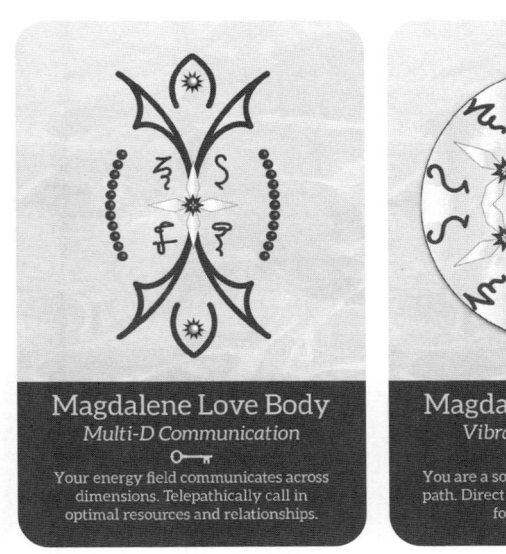

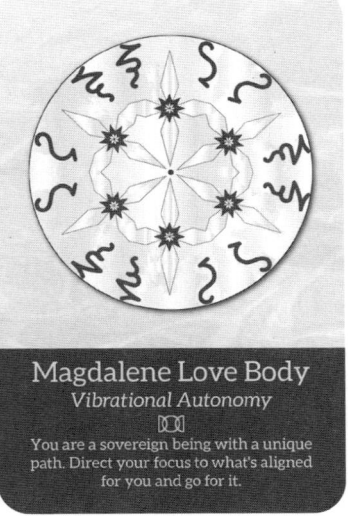

Magdalene Love Body
Multi-D Communication
Your energy field communicates across dimensions. Telepathically call in optimal resources and relationships.

Magdalene Love Body
Vibrational Autonomy
You are a sovereign being with a unique path. Direct your focus to what's aligned for you and go for it.

The Magdalene Love Body enhances your direct connection with divine love and union with Source, enveloping your creations with an energetic field, a body of love. This love body acts as an interface that is compatible with high vibrational experiences such as phenomenal abundance, and states of being such as grace, compassion, and union with Source.

The love body is connected to high levels of energy adeptness such as bilocation: being physically located in one place while being energetically present in another. This manifests as appearing to others in dreams, visions, and/or telepathic communication, which are genius-level capacities when it comes to manifesting without overdoing things. The Magdalene Love Body cultivates a greater sense of coherence within yourself as a potent spiritual being, which amplifies your presence and positive impact on the planet.

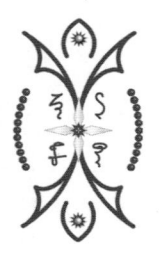

MAGDALENE LOVE BODY KEY
Multi-D Communication

> Your energy field communicates across dimensions.
> Telepathically call in optimal resources and relationships.

Your creations are Love Conceptions, alive, dynamic, ever-evolving, unique beings with universal intelligence. This code recognizes a very key component of the multi-D manifestation process—which can happen at any and all of these points—conception, development, birth, or full fruition. This constitutes the awareness that the love body is fully formed and anchored on all planes and dimensions. When you place your attention on the field surrounding you, emanating from your heart and your unique signature energy, you recognize that this energetic body actually builds to a point that it has a corporeal form. Your manifestations also have an energetic presence, a love body.

This form is vibrationally autonomous and can be felt, seen, and experienced across the globe. The love body is key to telepathic communication, bilocation, and sending wisdom in dreams and visions to others. When your creations build their energy—and Orgasmic Creation assists with this building of energy—the Magdalene Love Body is formed. At this point, the presence of the creation is pulsing strongly, continues to grow, and is highly magnetic.

Let's say your creation is a business entity—a separate, distinct, vibrationally autonomous being from you. When enough love builds in the business it begins to be its own vortex that is calling to it the optimal individuals, opportunities, and financial flow necessary for it to thrive. There is congruence and presence that emanates into the vibrational network of pathways that is key to manifesting while you sleep. In this you use energy, not effort.

This card invites you to commune with the Magdalene Love Body of your creations regardless of what developmental stage of consciousness they're in. Visualize your creations being enveloped in love and being radiant, coherent, and pulsing with the raw energy of creation. The Magdalene Love Body and all the codes are creation codes. The Magdalene Love Body is a love technology of wholeness and one that creates magical experiences and synchronicities, especially when you rest, meditate, and sleep.

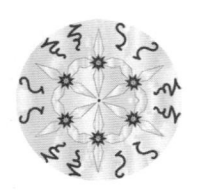

MAGDALENE LOVE BODY HOLOGRAM
Vibrational Autonomy

> You are a sovereign being with a unique path.
> Direct your focus to what's aligned for you and go for it.

Every line of a hologram contains the totality of that hologram. The Magdalene Love Body hologram is an environment that houses units of consciousness of highly refined vibrations, one in which you and your creations and those who come into contact with you are steeped in love. The Magdalene Love Body opens a wider reach, a greater global impact that goes beyond time and space. The vibrational signal that is essential to all actualization is broadcast loud and clear.

This card assists you in unhooking from outdated ways of being, such as having one foot on the brake and one on the gas or comparison, competition, and self-deprecation. It supports you in shifting any internal conflicts between two essential aspects of you, for example, being highly spiritual and incredibly wealthy. This way all your strengths are working together in a very congruent and synergistic way. You are unique and your path is unique to you. This code supports you in reconciling inner incoherence, enabling you to return to a state of grace and coherency between you and you.

When this code comes into your creation vortex, notice if

you have left your center, your home zone, your sweet spot, and if so, come back to your coherent nature. You are unique and connected to all that there is. You're in a state of individualized oneness, vibrationally autonomous without any confusion around what is yours to be, do, and have—and what isn't. You are clear on your direction and willing to be your own best guide.

Surrounded in the loving embrace of the Magdalene Love Body there is a deep stillness and divine knowing. Patterns such as people pleasing, trying to fit in, doing something out of obligation melt away. This code is all about spiritual mastery wherein you are following the path of your highest evolution, no matter how odd it may appear to others. Stop pretzling yourself and unfurl your Magdalene wings into your most loving, awake, present self.

This is also seen and felt in your creations on all levels. These creations radiate love and are beacons of wholeness, potently surrounded by love. Any droplet of lack is catapulted into another dimension for it cannot exist in the presence of this level of Source love. The Magdalene Love Body is Source love as an embodied presence.

APPLICATION

When you draw this card, soften your focus from the physical form of your creations to take in the presence of this manifestation. If it is your business, a book, money, a new home, a strong and healthy body, or a loving relationship, rather than seeing the physical form of the book or home, tune into the body of love that surrounds it. Tune into the presence of wisdom and clarity that envelops it. This accelerates all your creations, not only the one you are focusing on in this moment.

17
Embodied Radiance

"I am glowing with ever-growing energy."

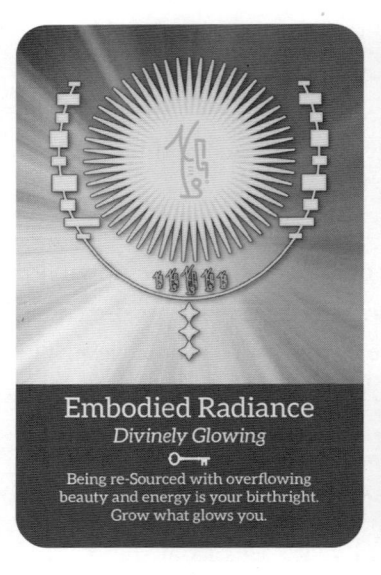

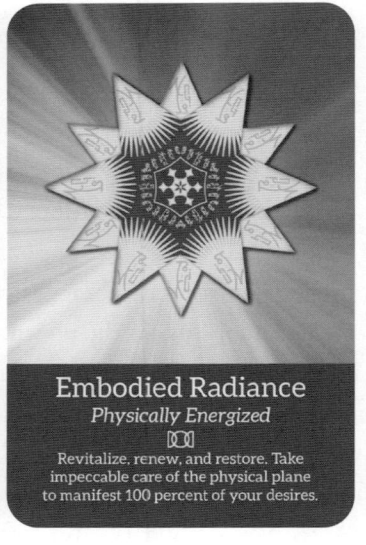

Embodied Radiance
Divinely Glowing
Being re-Sourced with overflowing beauty and energy is your birthright. Grow what glows you.

Embodied Radiance
Physically Energized
Revitalize, renew, and restore. Take impeccable care of the physical plane to manifest 100 percent of your desires.

Embodied Radiance naturally aligns your system to embody greater quotients of high vibrational energies, such as health, vitality, and those of your higher self. Your embodied love being self is highly magnetic and radiant. This code supports you in widening your reach as your love and physical stamina expand. Your attractor factor grows and you create stabilized expansion without the wobble, the push-pull, or the expansion-contraction.

As a creator being with the code of Embodied Radiance, all that you are aligned with turns to you like a sunflower to the sun. The radiant health, bountiful energy, dream house, the beloved, perfectly matched soul family, aligned partnerships, financial flow, creativity, a fantastic mood, or whatever matters most to you turns toward your energy because there is a vibrational match. You recognize the vibrational radiance of what you are looking for and vice versa. The highest path on your highest timeline magically unfolds before you and you naturally embody and physicalize your deepest desires.

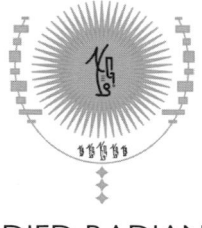

EMBODIED RADIANCE KEY
Divinely Glowing

Being re-Sourced with overflowing beauty and energy is your birthright. Grow what glows you.

You are naturally radiant and your energy glows. As you create, your energy glows even more. Your attractor factor and magnetism skyrocket. Your Embodied Radiance is the radiance that comes from the embodiment of your divine self, love body, and soul. By using the Magdalene Codes deck the units of consciousness of love in your system go up. You are vibrating at a higher frequency and speed. This renounces the previous habits and patterns you may have had in place, such as dimming your light, or frequently being tired, or having low energy. When you get out of the way of your natural radiance your glow bubbles up to the surface.

This card steps forward with a fierceness, guiding you to say no to anything and everything that doesn't enhance your energy. This doesn't mean you have to radically make over your life from one day to the next or necessarily change anything on the external planes. It means being fierce with the thoughts, emotions, and habits that drain your energy. You may declare the following statements to assist this shift: "Here where I reside is beauty. Here where I reside is divine order. Here where I reside is the radiance of the love of Source."

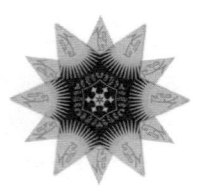

EMBODIED RADIANCE HOLOGRAM
Physically Energized

> Revitalize, renew, and restore. Take impeccable care of the physical plane to manifest 100 percent of your desires.

All the codes enhance your physical vitality, health, and Radiant Energy. This code does that in a primary way by supporting your embodiments to be strong. The strength of the container of your physical form, your body, and the containers your manifestations take—your home, career, relationships, finances—come from light and love. What you associate as strength is actually resonance, coherence, alignment, and stability. This stability is a natural capacity that the Embodied Radiance Code of Love adds to your manifestations so that you naturally expand, stabilize quickly, and then expand again.

Most of the time when you slow down your manifestations it's because there is a belief that you won't have enough energy or that you will burn out. This can occur when you are solely relying on your personal energy and action. Your personal energy is yours and yours alone, to be used only by you in a closed-circuit system within the space you occupy. The energy you circulate with others is infinite energy. Embodied Radiance restores the right relationship with the divine order of energy and recognizes that your radiance and glow is a contribution to all.

When you draw this card, you're encouraged to consolidate your energy to that which is essential. You may notice individuals, activities, or things naturally falling away as you attune to an even greater state of joy. This prioritization of your radiance and joy as top on your list may have come from a healing crisis or from your inner knowing. Don't be alarmed when things fall away. Simply lean into that which is emerging, revel in the space that has been opened up, and give thanks for what has been.

Rest, renew, rejuvenate. Taking impeccable care of the physical plane cultivates your capacity to manifest 100 percent of your desires. You are applying being a magical creator on the physical plane, and the field of creation responds in turn. Tune in. Are you called to exercise your body, dance, eat nourishing foods, meditate? Is now the moment to put systems in place, organize your home, or take a vacation? The new paradigm is no longer aligned to manifest anything that isn't aligned for you. Multi-D Abundance is what matters most to you. Lean into your natural beauty, your glow and your radiance, and watch gorgeous experiences rush in.

APPLICATION

When experiencing an expansion, fully take it into your body by breathing it in. If you receive money, breathe the money in. If you win an award, inhale the recognition. If you say no to something, rather than falling into people pleasing, breathe that win in. Revel in it, bask in it, be with it, allow it to integrate and consolidate in your system. This amplifies your energy and naturally begins to radiate out a more expanded presence. If you have a gift to give to someone, don't be attached to the outcome of your gift giving. Instead you simply place it on the altar for them to pick up or not.

Your Embodied Radiance is simultaneously close to your body and also knows no bounds; as a Magdalene manifester you are adept in creating through energy, the quantum field, and beyond time and space. Practice manifesting a goal that feels like a stretch or calling to you something that is physically located farther away from you. This way you are playing with nonlocality where your energy and the energy of what you are actualizing are in communion across distance or perceived size. This shifts the illusion lie that manifesting something "big" or far away, like a retreat center in New Zealand when you live in Florida, is more challenging than something "small" or doable that is right in front of you, like a parking spot. This is an illusion; your creations are actualized from far and near all the time. Perhaps what will create an even deeper Embodied Radiance in your system is someone or something that comes from the other side of the globe. This may be a product, mentor, or food. With both Star Love and Emerald Love, what deeply nourishes you and your projects may come in an unusual form, like the love you have from an animal, or wisdom from an off-planet lifetime, or a primary partnership with a guide.

Grow in what glows you.

18
Heart-Sentience

"I am guided by the higher knowing of my heart."

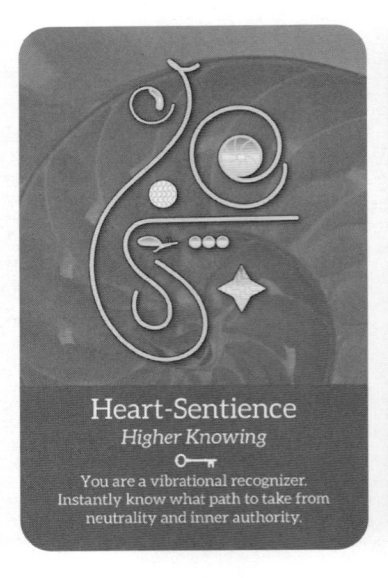

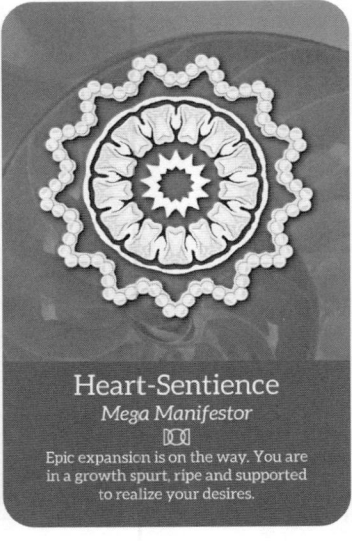

Heart-Sentience
Higher Knowing
You are a vibrational recognizer. Instantly know what path to take from neutrality and inner authority.

Heart-Sentience
Mega Manifestor
Epic expansion is on the way. You are in a growth spurt, ripe and supported to realize your desires.

Heart-Sentience is an irrevocable knowing, a coherent form of communication. It's a laser quick guidance system. This code supports you in making aligned decisions from your higher knowing, with adeptness. When you communicate heart-to-heart in a coherent energy the circulation of love between you and others expands. This is a path of enlightenment or enlovenment, where you hold, transmit, and circulate higher states of consciousness as a given.

Wherever you go, more love is created. The entire conversation of "Am I worthy? Do I deserve it?" dissipates. You're tapped into your vibrational recognition guidance system, which is a mega manifestation tool—a supercharged power to create expansive results. Inherent in Heart-Sentience is deep attunement to the divine order and well-being that naturally resides in the universe. It is a choice and a stance to create from a place of non-attachment while deeply knowing that the universe has your back and things are always working out for you for the highest and greatest good of all. We often speak of this elevated consciousness as creating from a place of "all is well, now what?" Which is very different then something is wrong that needs to be fixed or lack-based consciousness of something being missing. Instead you start your creation from a place of wholeness and knowing that all is well and you continue creating from that set point. This way you can do what you know needs to be done, say what needs to be said, and be neutral or unattached to the outcome. This allows energy to circulate in magical and life-enhancing ways.

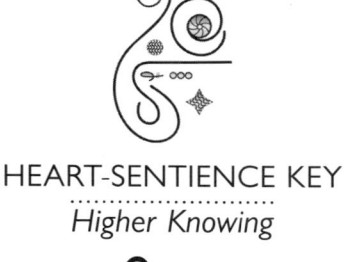

HEART-SENTIENCE KEY
Higher Knowing

You are a vibrational recognizer. Instantly know what path to take from neutrality and inner authority.

Your heart is the epicenter of circulation in your system and your heart chakra is one of the most highly receptive energy centers you have. As a new-paradigm creator you have outgrown the old ways of making decisions and navigating your world. This involved weighing pros and cons and leading primarily with your logical mind. Or inversely, perhaps you've been highly intuitive and have made decisions based solely on intuition and thrown logic out the window. This code encourages an intuitive-logical alignment, accessing the best of both while expanding beyond this integration into Heart-Sentience.

Heart-Sentience is a divine capacity of higher knowing and guidance that taps into an extrasensory knowing of your heart. Your heart wisdom is aligned with your soul's highest path and takes into consideration the knowledge that all facets of you have to contribute. This includes your intuition and logical mind. Heart-Sentience is an aligned combination of all the "claires"—clairsentience, clairvoyance, claircognizance, clairaudience—and instantly weighs them from a place of nonattachment and neutrality of the heart. You can imagine this as being similar to how a computer can organize and analyze a large amount of data quickly.

This code invites you to leap beyond simply following the calling of your heart and your heart's desires—although these are beautiful steps in the new-paradigm direction—into creating from all dimensions of you. Heart-Sentience incorporates the totality of your being instantaneously. It is the unification of all higher wisdom you are tapped into, synthesized into a deep irrevocable knowing. It's a knowing that is evident and crystal clear, and bubbles up from the inner sanctuary of your heart, connected to the heart of Source.

This code supports you in reclaiming your discernment, inner authority, and empowered capacity to create your life based on the inner signals that are relevant to your path in this incarnation. This is an essential way of navigating new Earth and manifesting from the new paradigm of wholeness.

When this card comes into your life, take a few moments and drop into your heart, listen, choose, and be informed as to the important next step or decision. Then ask simply if it's aligned with you. Guidance, implementation; implementation, guidance: the experience of navigating your path this way as a vibrational recognizer is freeing. It frees up energy and time that had been used inefficiently by overthinking or being attached to the outcome, to be spent instead in ways that matter most to you.

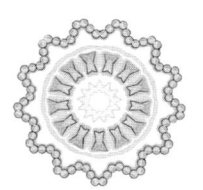

HEART-SENTIENCE HOLOGRAM
Mega Manifester

> Epic expansion is on the way. You are in a growth spurt, ripe and supported to realize your desires.

This code widens your bandwidth of receiving, having, and gifting from your heart to the hearts of others, making you a mega manifester and broadcaster of high vibrational wisdom. When you transmit energy from your Heart-Sentience, including all your communications with others and the universe, there is a palpable quality and synergy to your words and energy. Communicating your desires from your Heart-Sentience is potent—an invocation of truth and magic.

When you pull this card you are invited to broadcast your choices for the day and your manifestation spreads from the altar of the Heart-Sentience Code of Love. This wish, desire, or choice travels from your heart through the divine pathways of communication, directly to the heart of Source that then broadcasts through the divine pathways of communication to the altar of the heart of those whom your manifestation involves.

For example, if you are actualizing a relationship, whether it's with a friend, staff member, or becoming pregnant with a child, when you have this card as a part of your manifestation team your energetic signal goes out from your heart to the heart of Source. It's broadcast directly through the highest communication of heart coherence. When this happens, the perfectly matched relationships are magnetized to you. When you meet the other individual, it's like you have known each other for a very long time and you are picking up a conversation where you left off.

With the Heart-Sentience Code on your manifestation team what you are transmitting as you lead, teach, and offer your gifts to others is received on a deeper level. Life is about the hearts you touch. Allow this code to open your heart more to communicate from the space of openheartedness and high heart wisdom.

Being a mega manifester is like being someone who is very fertile choosing to get pregnant, or planting seeds in nutrient-rich soil. When Heart-Sentience comes into your card spreads it means that you are in a growth spurt and there is a ton of support for your desires to come into form. You are on a path of expansion, and Heart-Sentience is a stabilizer of high vibrations so that you may continue to grow from a place of strength and stability. Receiving, sharing, and having are acts of strength. Circulating love is an act of strength. Be in the space of the Infinite Love Meridian with the Heart-Sentience and watch your life bloom.

APPLICATION

Heart-Sentience is a sacred geometry environment that holds space for the highest possible outcome and also a capacity to circulate heart communication. It helps you navigate your path as a mega manifester from deep knowing. Take a moment to meditate on the Heart-Sentience key and hologram beings and visualize them at the heart of your home, career, connection with Source, and manifestation altar to create coherence and boost all that you do with the highest energetic infusion of Source energy.

19
Multi-D Abundance

"I am re-Sourced."

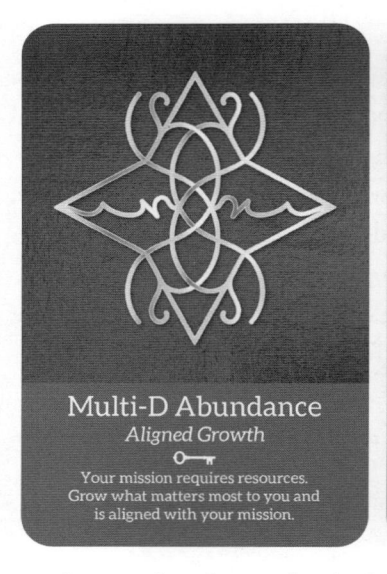

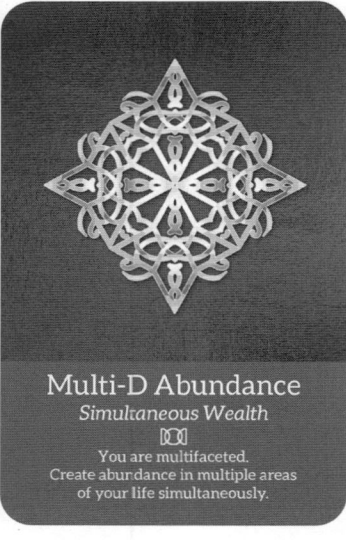

Multi-D Abundance
Aligned Growth
Your mission requires resources.
Grow what matters most to you and
is aligned with your mission.

Multi-D Abundance
Simultaneous Wealth
You are multifaceted.
Create abundance in multiple areas
of your life simultaneously.

Multi-D Abundance (multidimensional abundance) is the essence of living in the new paradigm of unity consciousness as a multidimensional being. A lot of what has been instilled in you by the collective consciousness imperatives is not relevant to your one-of-a-kind path in this lifetime. Stop making yourself wrong for being unique, different, and walking a path that absolutely has your name on it. When you stop trying to create it all—"all" meaning what everybody else deems important—and focus on what truly matters to you and your soul's path, magical things happen.

You're no longer bogged down by internal and external stuff that doesn't relate to you. You can integrate expansion quickly and stabilize the growth because it is natural for you. You can easily let go of old cycles and recognize that this makes space for what is to come. Union with Multi-D Abundance is a fulfilled, fruitful, and tailored life experience. It recognizes that some of the dimensions of your abundance are happening in the higher planes, during a dream state, when you're connected to your home star, and off-planet experiences.

If there is one code that has the potential to make the biggest difference in your life, it is this one. Get ready for the game changing, aligning, expansive support of Multi-D Abundance.

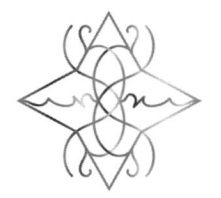

MULTI-D ABUNDANCE KEY
Aligned Growth

> Your mission requires resources. Grow what matters most to you and is aligned with your mission.

You are a multifaceted being and abundance is a multidimensional being. As you grow, the dimensions of your abundance grow. This code steps forward to gather your inner resources to inform and amplify your external resources. The time for more just for the sake of having more is outdated. The new paradigm is multidimensional, as is your abundance, determined by what your highest mission and path requires and what you truly desire. Simply stated, Multi-D Abundance is the cornucopia of resources you will create based on what matters most to you and what you are aligned with in many areas of your life.

This includes the four primary resources of Yummy Money, Sublime Time, Divine Relationships, Radiant Energy, and many more. Your purpose and the sharing of your gifts with others are forms of abundance. Learning, evolving, and growing are dimensions of abundance. Your relationship with Source and your higher self is a form of abundance. Moving your body, being in nature, community, creativity, beauty, material wealth that truly supports your highest vision, and internal assets are all dimensions of abundance.

This card reminds you that what you desire may actually come from focusing on another dimension of your abundance in conjunction with the one you are intentionally growing. For example, let's say you would like to have more financial abundance. In the old paradigm, you would put a lot of energy, focus, and action into building your financial abundance at the expense of other areas of your life. Your money goes up, however, your joy, energy, time with loved ones, self-care, health goes down. This is not abundance in wholeness, this is abundance in separation.

In order to circumvent the potential pitfalls of growing abundance in separation, it is important to nurture the entire ecosystem of abundance by going multi-D. Otherwise you may put the brakes on if you're not growing it in a way that nourishes the ecosystem that you reside in, the highest and best good for you, your clients, your family, and your community. Remember, what is good for you is good for others.

Multi-D Abundance is abundance in wholeness that honors your entire system and life. You don't just trade one form of abundance for another. Growing your financial abundance may actually flourish when you take more time to spend with your kids, in nature, or being creative. These areas of wealth may seem unrelated, however, they are interconnected. This code asks you to grow your abundance in alignment with what matters most to you. If learning makes you feel opulent then build time in your day to listen to podcasts, take a class, or try something new. If spending time in nature deeply satiates your nervous system and delights you, then be sure to make it a priority. If both these forms of abundance are a big part of your wealth temple then why not go for a walk and listen to a talk at the same time? This is an example of a multidimensional experience of Sublime Time where you are moving, in nature, and learning in simultaneity. There is also the abundance you experience in the higher planes while you are participating in an activity you enjoy, or spending time with those you love, including the nourishment that comes from non-bipedal relationships as with Emerald Love and Star Love.

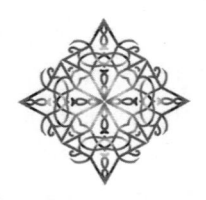

MULTI-D ABUNDANCE HOLOGRAM
Simultaneous Wealth

> You are multifaceted. Create abundance in multiple areas of your life simultaneously.

Steep in the hologram of Multi-D Abundance, relax into the energetic environment that this code brings—that of opulence and coherent and expansive abundance. Give yourself permission to feel deeply nourished by what it is that you do have—both the material abundance and also the internal riches of your gifts and talents, consciousness, and the capacity to instantly drop into a state of gratitude. Abundance is a birthright and these codes build energetic containers and an abundance body for this birthright to be experienced not as an idea or spiritual belief but in your physical dimension.

When the core of the altar stone of your Multi-D Abundance is love, all areas of your life are imbued with love. Love is inclusive and multidimensional. This card is an indication that you are on the precipice of radically shifting your internal experience to one of wholeness, and your external experience to embody abundance in a more coherent and aligned way.

Make a list of the top five areas of abundance that are important to you and your soul's mission. Notice where you may have been operating from a place where having all five felt like a stretch. Become aware that all these areas are interconnected dimensions of the abundance that your lifetime and mission require.

Notice where you may not have been giving yourself permission to want what you want or to prioritize something that may seem unrelated to your overall growth plan. Bring this area higher up on the priority list and be open, for it may not be what you thought it would be. Be willing to navigate your journey of Multi-D Abundance from a place of openness, receptivity, and exponential yet aligned growth, which will be sustainable and natural to expand again.

APPLICATION

Write down five forms of abundance that matter to you and your soul's mission. Now visualize these all being a part of one home or abundance body. They are not separate containers of abundance, but interconnected. Add these aspects of abundance as light beings to your manifestation team and ask these extensions of Source energy to communicate with you and to magnetize optimal environments, experiences, and opportunities.

20
Exponential Expansion

"I create exponential expansion, stabilize it quickly, and naturally expand again."

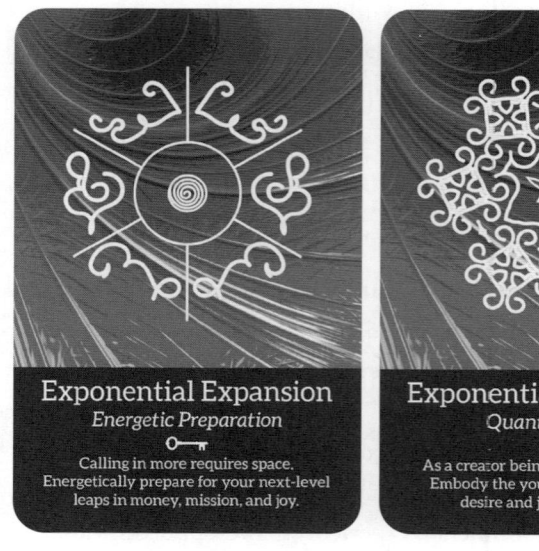

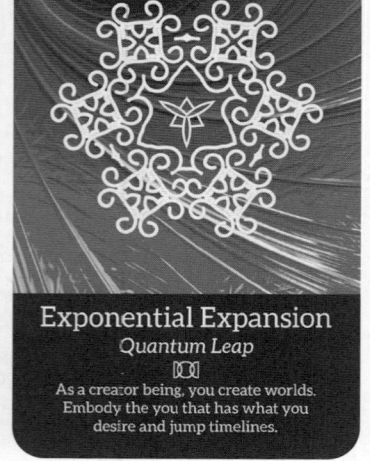

Exponential Expansion
Energetic Preparation

Calling in more requires space. Energetically prepare for your next-level leaps in money, mission, and joy.

Exponential Expansion
Quantum Leap

As a creator being, you create worlds. Embody the you that has what you desire and jump timelines.

Your growth is inevitable, a given. You are a divine being who is always evolving and expanding. Your abundance is a divine being who is always evolving and expanding. Exponential Expansion reminds you that expansion happens; it is a given. Know that expansion is so and so it is!

This paradigm shift from being hyper-focused on trying to *make* expansion happen into recognizing that expansion is happening all the time—it is a given—frees up your energy. Awareness of this opens you to the cocreative power of the universe and a divine partnership with your creation where expansion is simply a natural emanation of Source energy. Your energy and your creations shift from a place of your wondering if something specific is going to happen to it being a done deal, which opens up space for it to be so. Take a moment and notice the expansion that's already in your life. A lot of it was curated, consciously created, or cultivated, while some of it seemed to just happen. Regardless, expansion has occurred. It is natural. This code supports you in being even more conscious of your Love Conceptions and in curating them in a way that what is expanding is what you desire. And most of all, it places more of your attention on what happens after the expansion: the stabilizing factors. When you focus on stabilization as an essential and exponential part of the creation cycle you expand more effortlessly and frequently. This is an energetic secret that will skyrocket your manifestation success and the ease with which you receive and create.

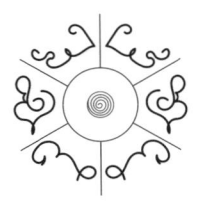

EXPONENTIAL EXPANSION KEY
Energetic Preparation

Calling in more requires space. Energetically prepare for your next-level leaps in money, mission, and joy.

Exponential Expansion is founded in fractal coherence and divine order. It is inevitable to expand and grow exponentially in a way that is absolutely natural for your system and your life. The old-paradigm illusion lie of the expansion-contraction hangover is probably something you've experienced. You have a win, a swoosh of money, promotion at work, meet the love of your life, move into your dream home . . . followed by a crash. This could be a crash in energy, getting sick, a breakup, a team member quits, you feel like you've done something wrong, or shame, doubt, or fear stops you in your tracks. These contractions are often spoken about as upper-limit symptoms. The higher purpose of the contraction is to stabilize the growth.

When you draw this key code you can flip this pattern on its head and build stable growth in as a part of the expansion. You anticipate the expansion and plan for it. You energetically prepare for it before it happens by creating a Magdalene Codes energetic altar with a card spread. You can call upon the love being that is Exponential Expansion to assist you in taking action to prepare for the expansion. If you know that you are going on a personal growth retreat or the trip of a lifetime or working with a mentor who is going to change your life, plan for that expansion. It can be as simple as painting your office so that when you come back from your retreat you have an external environment that honors and reminds your system that you've changed. It can be planning a day off after a big event to integrate, get a massage, read a book, go for a run, throw a dinner party, or whatever lights you up. It can also be solely on the energetic levels where you spend time getting your system used to the expansion by feeling it as if it's already here now.

This way, consolidation replaces contraction. It's important to stabilize your growth, to consolidate, streamline, and essentialize your actions and your expansions. This way the universal principle of fractal coherence is at play, where the leaves on a tree grow in a fractal, repeating pattern that is aligned and stable for the entire tree. There is an order to the expansion; a cycle to it that's natural. Sometimes the tree may require some support like a stick as it's first growing; however, most of the time the roots have already been stabilized to support the outer growth. With this Magdalene Love Being on your manifestation team, get ready to expand and then expand again without the crash, expansion hangover, or contraction.

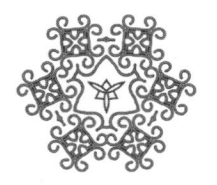

EXPONENTIAL EXPANSION HOLOGRAM
Quantum Leap

> As a creator being, you create worlds. Embody the you that has what you desire and jump timelines.

The difference between one and a million is zeros. The Exponential Expansion hologram code focuses on the exponential growth that is available to you. You are a multidimensional creator, creating beyond time and space. Thus you aren't bound to incremental growth of say a 10 percent improvement or linear 3D timelines. When this code comes into your manifestation spreads you're primed for a quantum leap. Lean into the current resources you have in your life and see where dormant potential is ripe to be realized. Identify containers of abundance wherein you can receive more without doing more.

For example, if you are a coach, author, or spiritual practitioner and you offer a group program that is positioned to have ten, one hundred, one thousand, ten thousand, or more individuals in it and it currently has five clients in it, there is space for you to receive more clients without doing more. Let's say you will coach those in your group once a week for two hours; whether you have five clients or one hundred, you will still spend that same two hours with your group. So there is space in that group container to expand without taking extra time for you to provide the service. Or if you're an author, having more individuals read your book doesn't take more time from you to deliver your gifts because the book can be read across the globe by thousands of individuals at the same time. Expanding the number of souls your books and programs reach and transform already quantum leaps the impact you are having. When you also contemplate the lives that these individuals touch, the ripple effect is exponential.

Where do you have potential for exponential growth that isn't being realized? This code supports you in aligning your energy system to quantum leaps; developing exponential growth in the way by which you stabilize the growth and keep expanding.

APPLICATION

Gaze at the glyphs and as much as possible affirm in your system that expansion is natural. Tap into the essence of the expansion, consolidate your efforts, streamline your actions, and compound your results. Less is more and more is less. Be in the zone of what brings you the greatest joy, and after every expansion, stabilize it.

21
Source Union

"I am one with the Source of all my Multi-D Abundance creations."

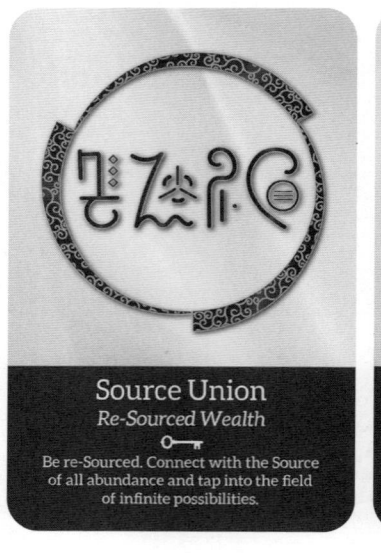

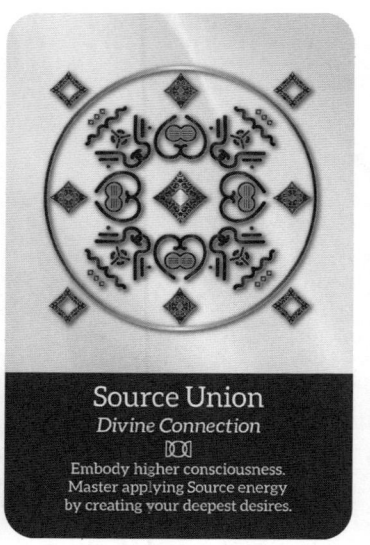

Source Union
Re-Sourced Wealth

Be re-Sourced. Connect with the Source of all abundance and tap into the field of infinite possibilities.

Source Union
Divine Connection

Embody higher consciousness. Master applying Source energy by creating your deepest desires.

Source Union magnificently positions you to be in the new paradigm of unity consciousness—fully tapped into the multidimensional energetics of abundance in wholeness, in individualized oneness. Your energy creations and your physical creations are one. Your ideas, inspirations, and the actualization of them are one. Your internal vibration is aligned with the frequency of what you are creating.

Abundance is moving at a faster vibration than lack. Source energy is moving at a higher vibration than separation consciousness. To embrace this code is to embrace a choice to live in union with your origin, your authentic self, with what matters most to you, and to be in an active state of self-love. It means to stand in the yoke of the Divine as an extension of Source energy. Source Union is your capacity to be in union with the source of abundance, which is Source. It means being in union with the source of love, money, time, energy, radiant health, partnership, creativity, divine order, and all that you connect with.

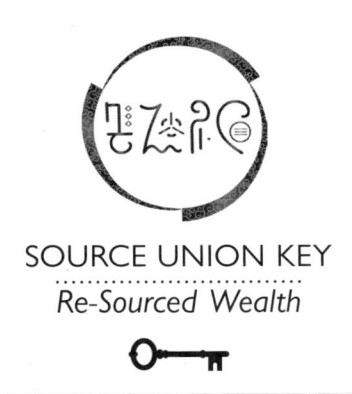

SOURCE UNION KEY
Re-Sourced Wealth

> Be re-Sourced. Connect with the Source of all abundance and tap into the field of infinite possibilities.

All of the light beings of your Love Conceptions as well as the units of consciousness of any resource originate from and is an extension of Source. Source refers to the Divine, God, Goddess, Great Spirit, All That There Is, and "source" as in origin. The origin of a body of water. The source of a creation. The source or origin of a unit of consciousness of abundance is Source. The monies you have in your bank account are units of consciousness of money. Money is a love being and money comes from Source. The source of money is Source and it flows to you through others.

Resources are beings of love with unique purposes and an overlighting deva or higher self. There is an overlighting deva of time, of money, of energy, and of relationships that is connected to Source energy. For example, if you have rosemary in your garden, that rosemary is connected to its origin, which is the rosemary species. The love being of rosemary is connected to Source. When you receive rosemary or harvest it from your garden you can send a wave of appreciation to the overlighting deva of all rosemary, to the source of rosemary. This connects you to abundance in oneness.

This appreciation practice deepens your relationship to the rosemary being of love and expands your consciousness from a place of limitation (the rosemary in your garden) to one of surplus (all rosemary on the planet and the rosemary deva). Let's say you receive money from a client, family member, or your job. In the old paradigm you narrow your awareness of the infinite supply to thinking that money only comes from that limited source. You misidentify that individual as your source, rather than being in the expansive truth of Source being your source. When you deeply appreciate the vessel the resource comes through—the client, family member, or job—while being connected to the infinite supply of the origin of that resource, you open up in beautiful ways.

Perhaps you are an empath and unconsciously you closed down receiving from others because you didn't want to be indebted to them or feel their anxiety or stress. With this code you can breathe deeply and know that there is an infinite supply of Source energy running through the money, love, or rosemary (for example) that you have in your life. This also shifts any outdated overlays that suggest that material wealth isn't spiritual for you, for you have become conscious that the source of all comes from the Divine.

When this key card comes onto your manifestation altars it is an invitation to be re-Sourced, to open wider, and to expand your wealth energetics to infinity and beyond. It means coming into a greater connection with the infinite supply and being in oneness with what you desire. The journey and the destination are seeded from the wellspring of Source energy. Watch how a sense of peace, neutrality, and expansiveness come into your projects.

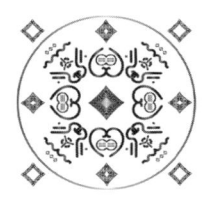

SOURCE UNION HOLOGRAM
Divine Connection

> Embody higher consciousness. Master applying
> Source energy by creating your deepest desires.

As a Magdalene Manifester you are employing the unseen and energetic realms to create on the physical plane, including Source energy and the highly inclusive energy of love. Being in union with Source energy in all now-moments is a highly attractive stance and vibration. You are naturally rearranging the universe to bring to you all the components required to manifest your deepest desires. Whether you desire a consistently high-vibe emotion as you go through your day, like appreciation or peace of mind, or a physical manifestation like owning your home free and clear, when you are connected to Source every day, life gets a lot more fun and abundant. For that which you are seeking comes to you with greater ease. Rest in the silent embrace of your Source connection, be in a state of oneness in your system—in union and self-love with self and all that there is.

Union is being in the same vibrational location with an energy, physical manifestation, or state of being. This card recognizes that your consciousness is one of your greatest areas of wealth. Your capacity to be in a coherent state with your origin, higher self, and connection to the Divine supports you in dropping resistance. When resistance and overlays are included back into wholeness you are available for the present moment to inform you as to next steps, to see the synchronicities that are all around you, and to be in a state of positive expectation that of course your creations will come to full fruition.

It is so and so it is!

This card is a pathway to connect to your most adept and realized enlightened and enloved self on an ongoing basis. Be connected to Source every day, and have this union be non-negotiable in all that you do. Separating from yourself and Source isn't loving to you or anyone else. When you are in union with Source you are at the top of your game, all in with your choices while being unattached to what unfolds. "This or something better" is the sweet spot of accelerated actualizations.

APPLICATION

When abundance comes into your life, send a wave of appreciation to the source of that abundance. If you are choosing to actualize clients and you would like to have ten clients and one shows up, send a wave of appreciation to that individual and to the source of aligned clients. When money comes into your life, send a wave of appreciation to the source of all money. When you are in a surplus moment (which is all moments) take a moment to send a wave of appreciation to the source of that abundance.

Once you get the hang of this and are on a roll with your appreciation, try this extra credit exercise. When you are in the presence of someone else's success, send a wave of appreciation and love to them and to the source of that abundance. This is especially potent if you find yourself in contracting, slower emotions like envy, comparison, and competition in the presence of others who have what you desire. When you're tapped into this higher perspective you are in an expansive state and naturally move away from perceiving things from a place of lack; instead, you choose to come from the abundance mindset and recognize there is more than enough to go around. Plus, it feels delicious to be genuinely happy for another's success and reaffirms with the universe that you are a yes for your own success, whatever that may look like to you, calling in your greater good with speed and ease.

22
Vibrational Visibility

"I shine brightly, drawing to me all that I desire and require with ease."

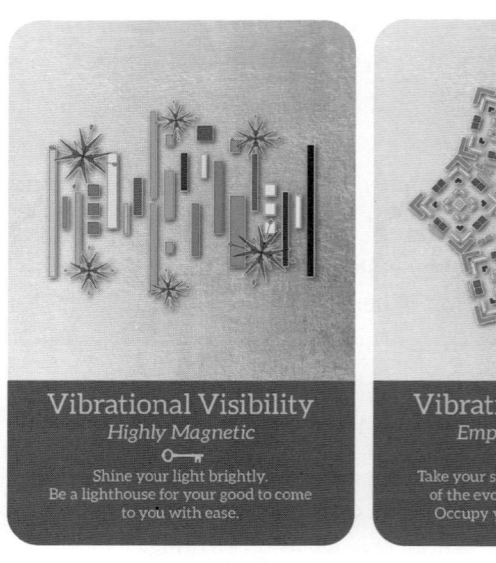

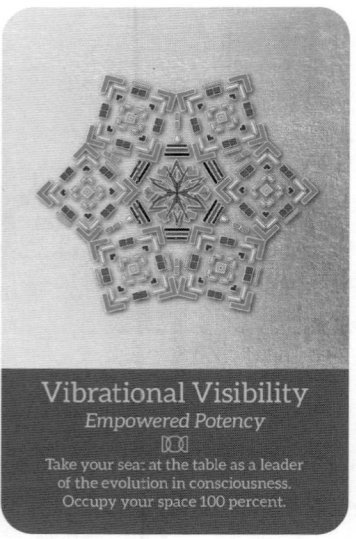

Vibrational Visibility
Highly Magnetic
Shine your light brightly.
Be a lighthouse for your good to come to you with ease.

Vibrational Visibility
Empowered Potency
Take your seat at the table as a leader of the evolution in consciousness.
Occupy your space 100 percent.

Vibrational Visibility is unapologetically shining the brilliant signature energy of the love being that is you and your manifestation. You are a vibrational being and it is your birthright to be seen, known, loved, and to be the love being that you are. Being vibrationally visible is a most empowered stance and seat at the table of unity consciousness. From this seat you allow, invite, encourage, beckon, and command that you are vibrationally visible to yourself and others.

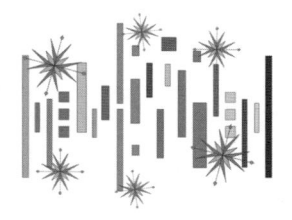

VIBRATIONAL VISIBILITY KEY
Highly Magnetic

> Shine your light brightly. Be a lighthouse for your good to come to you with ease.

This card steps onto your altar with prowess, potency, and an all-in attitude, inviting you to occupy your space 100 percent. It asks that you be visible to yourself, to be a lighthouse to others and your Multi-D Abundance. Vibrational Visibility of your signature energy acts like a master key of your life that positions you to have the unique experiences your mission requires. This increase in your light quotient catapults you out of the dimension of the survival consciousness operating systems. These may be exemplified by behaviors such as putting your light under a bushel or developing a fear of losing love or of being ostracized. Instead, it propels you into multidimensional living.

It is your Vibrational Visibility first and foremost that sends this signal and makes you visible to perfectly matched experiences and individuals. This code reminds you that repeating another pattern of invisibility, holding back, or distorting your power won't garner anything more. You have a master's degree in these repetitive patterns. You know everything there is to know about them.

With Vibrational Visibility turned on you are visible to everything that you have been calling to you. Often right as something is about to manifest and physicalize in the dimension where you can see it, touch it, feel it, and account for it in your bank account, the old-paradigm safety mechanism turns off the Vibrational Visibility. This is like ordering something online. You've placed your order. You've paid for the order. It's on the way. It's about to arrive, and then you move and it doesn't find you.

Instead, be highly magnetic by steadfastly shining your light from conception—where you place your order with the universe—to physicalization, where you hold it in your hands. This code is a fierce ally on your manifestation altar. Take off the veils of your true self and shine brightly every step of the way to your manifestation. Watch the universe rearrange itself to support you and your creations.

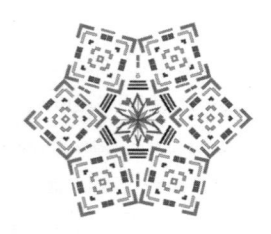

VIBRATIONAL VISIBILITY HOLOGRAM
Empowered Potency

Take your seat at the table as a leader of the evolution in consciousness. Occupy your space 100 percent.

Vibrational Visibility is an advanced manifestation technique wherein you turn up the volume of your signature energy in all the dimensions in which you reside. This makes you highly visible to your guides, optimal relationships, and resources. Plus, when you call in more abundance, Vibrational Visibility has a stabilizing effect because your growth is grounded and customized to your frequency, thereby creating an ever-unfolding expansion spiral. This way the time between your creations shortens. You expand and what you've created is easily integrated because it belongs to you and you alone. In this, your creations buoy your frequency, adding energy to you and your life, which then creates the next ascension spiral of expansion, and then the next.

This card creates an environment of empowered potency. Here, anywhere that you were sharing a diluted version of yourself or your gifts easily reverts back to the full potency of you. Being your full self is not only an empowered way to be, it expands your energy multidimensionally so you are connected to Source and the vastness of you. Bask in the full brilliance of your signature energy and that of your actualizations. Shine brightly and give permission to others to do the same. When you unleash the uniqueness of who you are into your projects and creations they are founded in a vibration that is true to you.

You always have the choice to share knowledge, your inner workings, and the deepest aspects of yourself with others on the physical plane—or not. You can choose to tell someone you are using a manifestation system that was downloaded from the Magdalenes or you can simply vibrate this in your field and model the evolution you create for yourself. Vibrational Visibility does not mean that you stop being at choice as to what you show or share on the physical plane. It actually means that you are more discerning than ever and the octaves of you are vibrating at their full frequency in the dimensions where they are most optimal. If it's aligned for you to not share something, make this choice from a place of knowing, not hiding.

When you operate multidimensionally and your creations are visible in many dimensions and someone comes into contact with them they will only tap into or see the vibrations they have vibrational access to and resonance with. This opens up a greater willingness in your system to no longer hold back and to shine brightly, and to see yourself, your creations, and others as what they are: love in form. Manifesting and new-paradigm living is not a one-size-fits-all experience. Be in the full potency of what is aligned for you and what you choose to be, do, and have, and let what isn't a perfect match for you zig while you zag.

APPLICATION

When you're called to accelerate the timeline of your creation coming into form, Vibrational Visibility is a key ally in your endeavors. Visualize your creation with the Vibrational Visibility glyphs and turn up the natural signature energy of your manifestation. Amplify the reach and visibility of your project to those who are looking for you and your creations. Attract and choose to come into contact with those who have a supportive role in the actualization of your manifestation. Being a diluted version of yourself slows things way down. Instead, turn up the volume of your frequency to full tilt boogie.

23
Fully Realized

"I am a manifestation master. All that I create comes to full fruition."

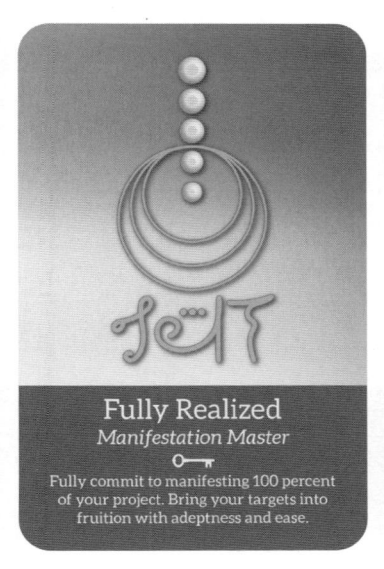

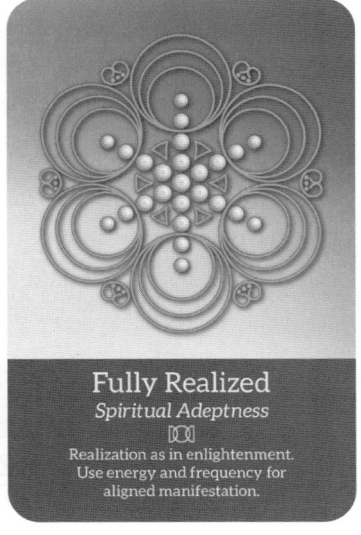

Fully Realized
Manifestation Master
Fully commit to manifesting 100 percent of your project. Bring your targets into fruition with adeptness and ease.

Fully Realized
Spiritual Adeptness
Realization as in enlightenment. Use energy and frequency for aligned manifestation.

The Fully Realized Magdalene being and new-paradigm manifesting code comes from the Fully Realized divine-verse beyond the central sun. The Earth and her inhabitants are moving into a higher frequency and are in the evolutionary stage in consciousness of becoming Fully Realized—realized as in fully embodying the higher consciousness of wholeness, realized as in going from the duality of always being separate from what you desire (lack, fear, doubt) to jumping into union with your desires (abundance, joy, love). This is a return to wholeness. As you joyously realize higher states of consciousness and your manifestations become realized, you play an essential role in accelerating this return of love beings on Earth.

This code creates an illusion-free zone of wholeness, grounding higher states of awareness. The Fully Realized energy is one that is consistent. It's permanent. It's there. Once the genie is out of the bottle, it doesn't go back in. Once you vibrate at a certain level of consciousness, that consciousness is part of you. It just is. When spiritual masters like you come to a certain level of realization, you don't revert back to the level of consciousness you had before. You integrate this leap in consciousness and abundance. You spend more now-moments being Fully Realized, as a given set point dialed into higher consciousness.

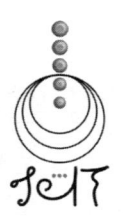

FULLY REALIZED KEY
Manifestation Master

> Fully commit to manifesting 100 percent of your project.
> Bring your targets into fruition with adeptness and ease.

You are in a constant state of becoming, as are your creations. As you manifest, your creations become realized. Consistent, predictable realization of 100 percent of your creations is a skill set, choice, and practice, one that takes energetic and physical plane commitment. This code stepped into your field today to ask one important question. Are you fully committed to creating 100 percent of your project or have you slid into a default position of creating 80 percent or 50 percent or x percent of your desire? There isn't a right or a wrong answer here, simply awareness. Shine the light anywhere you may not have been all in on bringing your manifestation into its possible highest expression. And choose again.

Perhaps you've been holding back out of a fear that having 100 percent of your desires every time will mean something about you that it actually doesn't mean. For example, that you will be alone, perceived as greedy, or that you won't be able to handle the expansion. Tap into the universal truth that it isn't harder for Source to create 100 percent of something (for that is its natural state) than 80 percent of something. Notice the energy that gets freed up when you know your manifestation is a done deal. Decide that it is already done. See, feel, know, and taste it being Fully Realized now.

Being Fully Realized eliminates the wobble, indecisiveness, and doubt, and returns you to your original spark of inspiration in which crossing the threshold was a given, an absolute, an is-ness. This code reminds you that your creation is already Fully Realized in the multidimensional planes and now the fun part is simply living into it in a way where you build the experience of consistently and predictably manifesting 100 percent of your desires on the physical plane. Fully Realized—not half-baked or partially created—full fruition.

You've got this!

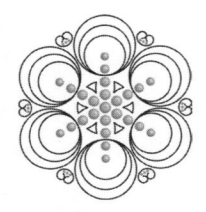

FULLY REALIZED HOLOGRAM
Spiritual Adeptness

> Realization as in enlightenment. Use energy and frequency for aligned manifestation.

Being Fully Realized speaks to crossing a threshold that once it is crossed it's fully inhabited and created. The tadpole becomes the frog; your states of higher consciousness are fully anchored and embodied. Realization as in enlightenment, adeptness, and being fully awake. This hologram code holds an environment for you to fully embody your higher states of consciousness as a given. It's asking you to shift out of the yo-yo, up-down states of waking up and going back to sleep or knowing a spiritual truth and then popping out of it, into integrating your higher consciousness in more now-moments.

Being in a state of higher consciousness and having your creations broadcast this higher consciousness supports your creations in being more fulfilled and alive. You're here to experience and play full-out, to have your hands in the clay as a creator without pushing, overworking, or frenzied action to make up for a lack of alignment. Rather you are a manifestation master. Your creations have a divine plan, an innate intelligence to be birthed onto the Earth Star at this time. This card supports you in being the being that creates your dreams with ease.

When you manifest from this code you are conscious in your choices, aligned in your intention, and on a path of illumination. This creation code is the universal principle that all that there is exists in each and every moment, so the full realization of your creations exist. This code amplifies your spiritual adeptness in using a higher consciousness and frequency to create. Leveraging higher states of awareness is a fast track to create consistently and predictably.

Your action is a very small percentage of what creates worlds and your Love Conceptions. This code enhances your spiritual adeptness, your higher consciousness, your enlightenment. Enjoy the higher states of knowing and multidimensional awareness and allow them to inform your creations. If things aren't working out, try and get some insight from a higher perspective, for there is a deeper reason for this, a message. Is it time to redirect? Is something better emerging or are you being guided to keep going with a fierce knowing that it is already done?

APPLICATION

Gazing at the Fully Realized glyphs with your Love Conception in mind we invite you to feel into 10 percent of your manifestation being realized, then 20 percent, then 30 percent. Notice your sensations. Do you feel safe? Is it exciting? Keep going from 40 percent all the way to 100 percent full fruition, noticing which percentage feels like a done deal and where things start to feel wobbly, if at all. Practice being with the 100 percent Fully Realized state of your creations to prepare your system energetically for them to come into form. What you seek and desire is on its way to you!

24
Magdalene Love Being

"I am an ambassador for love."

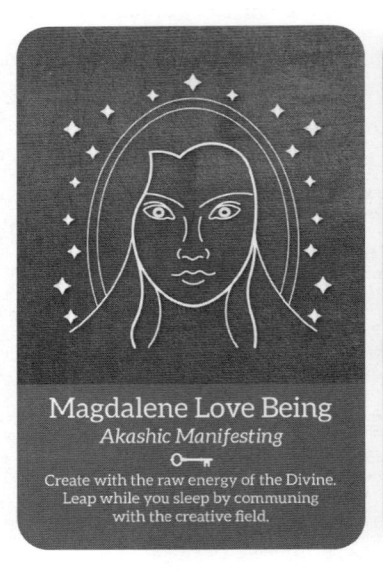

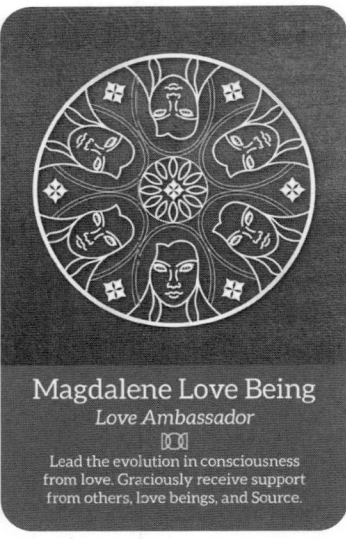

Magdalene Love Being
Akashic Manifesting
Create with the raw energy of the Divine. Leap while you sleep by communing with the creative field.

Magdalene Love Being
Love Ambassador
Lead the evolution in consciousness from love. Graciously receive support from others, love beings, and Source.

You are a Magdalene Love Being. Your Fully Realized Love Conceptions are Magdalene Love Beings. Your Multi-D Abundance is a Magdalene Love Being. You are beloved. Being an ambassador of love, an akashic manifester, and a vibrational leader is a charge, quest, or higher purpose that propels you to create for the joy of it. This code supports your system in getting all the oars rowing in the same direction, consolidating your energy, opening your heart, and guiding your focus so that you're resilient and aligned. Your words, deeds, and success matters, and your vibration underneath all of those is key to their manifestation. Imbue your manifestations with love, and more love is created.

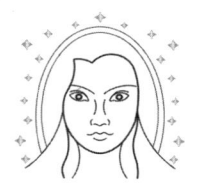

MAGDALENE LOVE BEING KEY
Akashic Manifesting

> Create with the raw energy of the Divine. Leap while you sleep by communing with the creative field.

As a Magdalene Manifester you have an innate resource, a magical genius, to create in the ambrosial hours, in the sublime supine position, using the horizontal plane and the energy of love. As you manifest while you sleep, you tap into the multidimensional creator codes of all creation—the Divine Ray,* also known as Akasha, the fabric of Creation. The creative field is always there while you sleep, and as you take aligned action you manifest multidimensionally. You are a Magdalene Manifester. You're following your own path. You're not getting pulled out of your center. You align energy, and form follows.

---

*The Divine Ray—the Oneness Ray connects you to the fabric of creation. See the guides' and my 2013 book *The Council of Light: Divine Transmissions for Manifesting the Deepest Desires of the Soul* to learn more about the Divine Ray.

Drawing this Magdalene Love Being Code is a sign it's time to turn up the volume on your magical capacity to leap while you sleep, to manifest through magic, the nighttime, the void, the energy of Akasha. Take back approximately a third of your Sublime Time to manifest while you sleep, and restore your birthright of multidimensional communication. Communicate in the higher planes with those individuals you are aligned with and who have key roles in your Love Conceptions.

Intend before going to sleep that you will receive your creations through the Magdalene Love Being Code. This code is a net, vessel, receptor site connected to your Magdalene Love Body, Magdalene Molecule, and your Magdalene Heart that fully turns on the magic in the love being that is your creation. Upon awakening, pay special attention to any insights you may receive. When you feel stuck as to how to proceed, take a nap, meditate, lie down, place the cards on your body, snuggle with a loved one, or commune with your guides. Yin in to win!

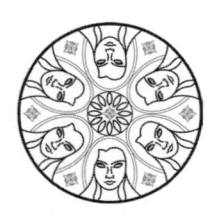

MAGDALENE LOVE BEING HOLOGRAM
Love Ambassador

**Lead the evolution in consciousness from love.
Graciously receive support from others, love beings, and Source.**

As your Love Conceptions come into form they become Magdalene Love Beings with the codes that have supported them in becoming Fully Realized. Your manifestations broadcast the energies of Ecstatic Bliss, Emerald Love, Vibrational Visibility, and more. They come into form with an energy body, a love body just like your system has.

This means that your creations have a hologram of energy around them that vibrationally stabilizes the physical expression in a way that is elevated. When you draw this card you are invited to bring what seems to be separate aspects of what you are creating, like teeth on an open zipper, together, like zipping up the zipper. This card is reminding you that any creation you desire, big or small, is absolutely do-able and be-able because you are supported and your creation is a love being. Rather than being overwhelmed you feel nourished; you move from feeling scattered to crystal clear, from exhausted to vital.

Remember that you also have a team of support on the higher planes, your manifestation council of love beings that these Magdalene Codes of Love are cocreating with you and the universe. This card encourages you to shift out of any "do it alone mentality" into opening to the support that is already around you. Ask your guides and at least one individual to assist you today. Make a request and notice what this brings up in your system. The new paradigm is marked by cocreation, collaboration, community, and creating win-win-win opportunities.

Your creation is connected to a higher vision and purpose. Clarify the desire underneath your desire and steep in your bigger *why*—why you are called to create it. How does it not only assist you, your loved ones, and your community, but also those whom you are a vibrational leader for in the global shift in consciousness. Tapping into your expanded vision fortifies your Love Conceptions and accelerates your path from inspiration to creation.

Be an ambassador of love.

APPLICATION

When you draw this card it is a great time to actively turn up your manifestation practice while in a being state—either lying down or while you are sleeping. Create altars that you place next to you while you are resting and sleeping. Intend that your sleep and rest are deeply nourishing to your system. Claim that you magically manifest through the yin energy of resting.

CARD SPREADS AND MANIFESTATION VORTEXES

※

We've shared the importance of focus when doing the card spreads. We have also identified that you are creating on the inner and outer planes, and we've invited you to widen your manifestation practice to include both. Now let's go into how to use this manifestation deck in more detail, including best practices, possible spreads, and cocreating more deeply with the resource codes.

How to Use the Card Spreads

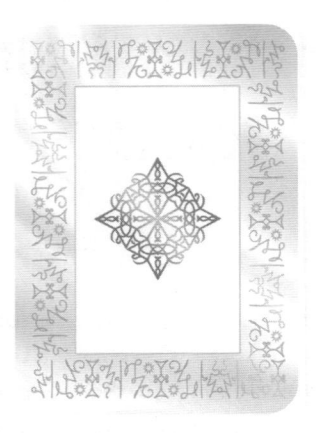

Back of the Cards

To begin your card spread choose your focus and the number of cards you are going to draw. Shuffle the cards and spread them out with the code side facedown, so the back of the card image you see on all the cards is the same as above. Hover your hand over the cards—use your nondominant hand to enhance your being state, openness, receptivity, and crystal clear guidance or use your dominant hand to amplify the creative empowerment of your commitment and the assured creative force and momentum that comes when you are all in on creating what you desire.

With your hand over the cards notice if you have a tingling in your palm, a feeling of yes this is the card to pull, hear specific guidance like "pull the eighth card from the bottom" or "this one" or whether there is another signal that guides you to a certain card. Alternatively, split the deck into two stacks. Choose a stack and then pull cards from the top or the bottom. Use your Heart-Sentience as to how you draw your cards, for each spread is as unique as are you.

Once you have the cards laid out in front of you take a moment to notice your first impressions or where your focus is attracted. A key element to building a living relationship with the codes is connecting with the signature energy of them as love beings. A primary way to do this is through your visual senses as you see the glyphs and take in words on the card and in this guidebook. Experiencing the codes through your eyes and optic nerve balances the left and right hemispheres of your brain and feminine and masculine energies.

Place the card spreads where you can see them—on your desk, night table, or mirror—in a type of altar. Do this to enhance your relationship to the multidimensional energy vortex your spread creates. You are in vibrational proximity to and basking in this high-vibe energy container. You may feel called to place an item related to your manifestation underneath or adjacent to your altar of cards. This can be a bank statement with the amount of money you're choosing to have in your account written onto it, or a photo of you doing something you enjoy—riding a horse, traveling, or spending time with your best friend. Or you may feel called to place a sacred object that holds special meaning to you, like a crystal or piece of jewelry, on top of the cards to amplify the energy vortex. When you pull a code, you may feel called to gaze upon the cards for a few minutes or several seconds.

Gazing at the sacred geometry shapes, trace them with your eyes or hand in the air. This deepens your connection with the glyphs. Imagine the symbols as multidimensional rather than being flat on the card. The hologram glyphs create holographic, multidimensional energy containers. The key glyphs unlock different energies in your timeline, life, system, and the dimensions of your abundance. The four resource codes amplify your abundance in four essential areas of money, time, relationships, and energy.

If called, place glyphs on or around your body in order to align with your desires. Receive mini energy sessions with the love being codes and the Magdalenes. You may be aware of energetic shifts within and without—always in alignment with your free will and conscious choice. Remember, you guide and direct the process, for you are a creator being.

Follow Your Inner Guidance

We provide several possibilities for energy vortexes that work incredibly well, and we invite you to tap into your inner guidance. Use the templates we've laid out and play with your own. These card spreads are alignment sessions with the Magdalenes and the codes. As you've learned, they create energy containers and energy vortexes. They are altars wherein your ideas and your inspirations can expand into form. They calibrate your system to a whole new way of manifesting in alignment with sacred union.

Enjoy these card deck spreads. Use your intuition in terms of the length of time that you keep them up. When any particular card is out of the deck it's not in play for you to use regularly. Again, there's no right or wrong. If you notice a fear of getting it wrong or trying to get it right, fold that back into the wholeness. The energy will run as long as your system requires even if you put the cards back in the deck or you keep them separate longer. There are higher principles at play here. Just have fun with it. This Magdalene deck is designed for expansion in a way that's natural for your system.

Enjoy!

ONE-CARD SPREAD
Daily Support

The one-card spread offers daily support and creates an energy vortex for the day or a segment of the day. Before choosing a card set your intention. Pose a question, request guidance, or ask for a theme. Invite the Magdalene being of the code that you draw to be with you. Receive inspiration, divination, or a message for the day.

Like a code of honor that you uphold, the code you draw in your one-card spread is a way of being you embody. Coming from this being state is a fast track to living in the new paradigm. If you pull Ecstatic Bliss, fold Ecstatic Bliss into your day. You may keep your planned activities while being in an internal state of Ecstatic Bliss. It may be a wink from the Divine to say, "I've pulled the Ecstatic Bliss card. Where can I add in lunch with a friend, a yoga class, or an experience that's going to be fun?"

TWO-CARD SPREAD
Feminine-Masculine Alignment

The two-card spread supports you in bringing the feminine and masculine energies into sacred union—to align being and doing. You may be called to this spread when you notice a pattern of overdoing to make up for lack of alignment, or overbeing, where you've done a lot of inner work yet aren't taking action.

Or this may occur when you notice a competing commitment. For example, you are committed to making an even bigger difference on the planet through your career. And you are committed to spending more time with your family. These commitments seem to be in competition with one another. As we have discussed previously, there may be a belief that if you have one it will be at the cost of the other. Remember, a core element of the Magdalene manifestation deck is Multi-D Abundance, which is not about trading one form of abundance for another, which perpetuates a state of scarcity. Instead, it's about expanding in a way that's stabilized and grows your wealth in multiple dimensions simultaneously.

This spread works beautifully to create internal alignment between two primary aspects of yourself that have been in conflict. Here are some examples: being a CEO and a mom, or being an introvert with a deep calling to transform the lives of thousands through public speaking, or being highly structured while working in a corporate environment and creating from flow as an artist, channel, or energy healer in your spare time. These may have been paradoxical or seemed to not go together in the past. The new paradigm of Magdalene beingness is to have all you desire in alignment with what is coherent for your unique path. It's not about having more for the sake of having more or having some of what you desire but not all of it.

When you notice you're in a frenzy of activity to make up for being out of alignment, it's a superlative time to recalibrate your masculine and feminine energies. Leaning too heavily on actions will slow things way down, for energetic frequency is what creates the bulk of your manifestations. Of course, you're going to be in action, utilize strategic thinking, and combine these with your energy alignment for this is what creates rapid actualization.

To begin, draw one card from the deck. Then search through the deck to pull the partner card of the first one. For example, if you draw the Infinite Love Meridian key glyph, look through the deck to find the Infinite Love Meridian hologram glyph. If you happen to pick a resource code, go through the deck and find a second resource code.

Once you have your two cards, hold them in front of your eyes, the key glyph in your left hand for the left brain and the hologram in your right hand for the right brain. Attune the hemispheres of your brain to work together as you gaze. When you feel complete, place them on your desk next to each other and gaze upon them as guided. Alternatively, you may move into a supine position with a card on the left and another on the right side of your body. Or place one on your spleen (lower left ribs) and the other over your liver (lower right ribs). As always, use your intuition as to what is optimal for you and your creations. You may be guided to switch it up and hold the key glyph in the right hand and hologram in the left. When you choose a resource code, use your Heart-Sentience to inform you as to where to place them. The two-card spread aligns the masculine and feminine energies, the internal and the external aspects in you and your creations.

THREE-CARD SPREAD
Manifest While You Sleep

The three-card spread—the trio of abundance spread—works phenomenally when you are in a supine position, lying down, resting, or before you go to sleep. You can position the three cards in a triangular shape, either an upward-facing pyramid or a downward-facing pyramid. In this you will have one card that is the apex of the pyramid and two cards next to each other. If you do this before sleeping put the cards on your nightstand, under your bed, or in three corners of the room. This creates a pyramid hologram that you will sleep within that calls to you what you require for that manifestation from the source of all abundance.

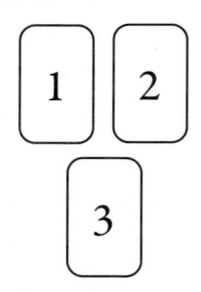

Three-Card Spread

The trio of abundance spread can be for manifesting one area of abundance, like a home, ideal clients, or a new career. It can be for one thing, or you can have a trio of abundance for three things under that subject of home, clients, or work. Let's say you're creating a Yummy Money altar for financial freedom. You can have a card for owning your home free and clear on one side of the triangle. Another side of the triangle would feature the aim of developing a six- or seven-figure business. The third side of the triangle is a net worth you have where your passive income exceeds your expenses. You can create this trio of abundance, this triangle of wealth. It's a Yummy Money altar with three Yummy Money objectives.

Then draw a card for each side of the triangle: one for owning your home free and clear, one for your annual income, and one for your net worth. The correlating Magdalene Code primarily supports that aspect of your Yummy Money triangle or pyramid. Again, this creates a vortex that you are sleeping within.

We chose three external expressions of Yummy Money. You can also amplify states of internal being. Decree that creating money is joyful. Decide that your experience with money is magical and nurturing. (See the Yummy Money Spreads on page 181 for more tips on enhancing your money relationship.)

Manifesting while you're sleeping and in a horizontal position is magical and a foundational key to the Magdalene Codes of Love manifestation deck and program. You're using your restorative, regenerating, and receptive state, your horizontal body, as a way of manifesting. This not only reclaims a third of your manifestation time (or however long you sleep), it also amplifies the aligned action you are taking, culminating in even better results. When your body is in a horizontal position with a relaxed focus—for example, lying down during the day, taking 15 minutes to do a trio of abundance spread—you are wildly receptive and highly magnetic. Knowing there is untapped creation potential while you sleep and in these mini-manifestation sessions gives you incentive to add them into your regular actualization practice.

The codes restore your feminine ways of manifesting. Then all you're doing in the masculine expression has the support of the sacred union of the two. Of course, you can draw three cards without lying down, and may find it beneficial to place the three cards side by side rather than in a triangle. However, we particularly recommend this trio of abundance, this three-card spread for manifesting while you're resting or meditating in a supine position and sleeping. Think of these energy vortexes and energy containers as an energy session with the Magdalene Codes.

FIVE-CARD SPREAD
Long-Term Projects

Use this card spread for a longer-term project like writing a book, getting pregnant, birthing and raising a child, remodeling a home, creating a thriving community, or strengthening your connection with Source. These projects have a longer trajectory or duration. Or use this spread for new ways of being or thinking, such as enhancing your mood, and/or generating supportive thoughts that are vastly different from the discouraging ones you've had.

Let's say overthinking, perfectionism, or the do-it-alone mentality have been a bottleneck to your successful manifestation practice. These patterns have been in place for a while, so having support to shift them and create new ways of being—such as enjoying peace of mind, completing projects without needing them to be perfect, and delegating to others—are ideal focuses for this spread. This energy vortex widens your bandwidth and gets you off the expansion-contraction roller coaster and onto a pathway of stabilized growth that you can integrate and embody in ways that are coherent for your system.

The five-card spread forms a cross with both a horizontal and vertical column. It can also be thought of as creating an energy container, casting a circle or sacred ceremony space for your manifestations to be supported. To generate this, call in the five directions of east, west, north, south, and center—or the five elements of Air, Fire, Water, Earth, and Akasha. Begin with the top card of your vertical column and pick the first card. Then draw a second card that will be for the middle. Then draw card number three for the bottom. Card number four will be to the left of your center card. Card number five is to the right. You've created a five-card spread.

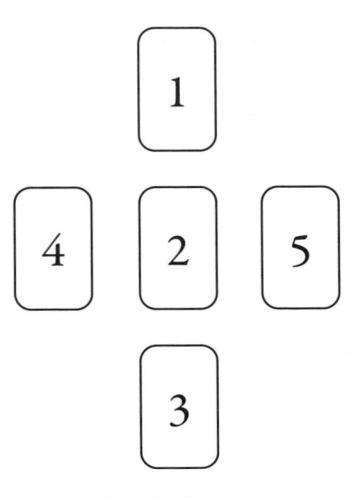

Five-Card Spread

WILD CARD SPREAD
Divinely Guided

Use your intuition to create the spreads that are aligned to you. Our central guidance is that there's no right or wrong way to do card spreads. We're providing some options, and we invite you to create a wild card spread based on what feels aligned for you in the moment.

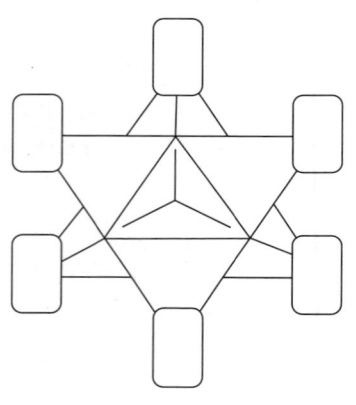

Star Tetrahedron Wild Card Spread

Draw four cards and place them in the corners of your room before you sleep. Pull six cards to form a diamond or star tetrahedron (as shown above), or multiple cards to create a sphere. Or use all the cards in the deck to create a sphere, or line them up horizontally across the couch. Perhaps you're in the mood to pull ten cards and place them around you or on your body while you take a nap. Maybe you're called to pull nine cards to create a square with three rows of three. Write down on pieces of paper nine things that you're choosing to manifest, and draw a card for each, like a bagua in feng shui. There are many possibilities. Use your divine guidance with the wild card spreads.

Resource Codes Spreads

You may feel called to create manifestation altars for a resource code wherein you dedicate your Love Conception altar to money, time, energy, or relationships. You can follow the above spreads and simply add a resource code. Let's say you're doing a manifestation spread for Divine Relationships. Go through the deck and pull out the Divine Relationships card. Then with that resource card as the primary purpose, proceed with a one-, two-, three-, five-, or wild card spread. You would have two cards if you are doing a resource code one-card spread: Divine Relationships plus the card you draw. In the two-card spread, you would have three cards, and so on.

Sometimes you may be guided to do a resource spread where you dial in on one resource code. Other times you can open the floodgates by focusing on two types of resources, like Yummy Money and Divine Relationships together. Money expansion requires more relationships and vice versa. You can pull one, two, three, or four resource codes for your manifestation altars and then choose as many cards as you would like to create an altar for these resources.

Go deeper into the four resource codes with the sixteen-card spread and the internal and external energy vortexes below.

180   Card Spreads and Manifestation Vortexes

SIXTEEN-CARD SPREAD
Create Multi-D Abundance

You could also do a spread for all four resource codes in the spirit of Multi-D Abundance. Here is a sixteen-card spread that is very powerful. To begin pull out the four resource codes and place them on top of your card spread side by side in a row of four. Then shuffle the deck and cut the cards in three stacks. Choose the stack that you are most drawn to and place it on top of the other two stacks, recombining the deck into one stack.

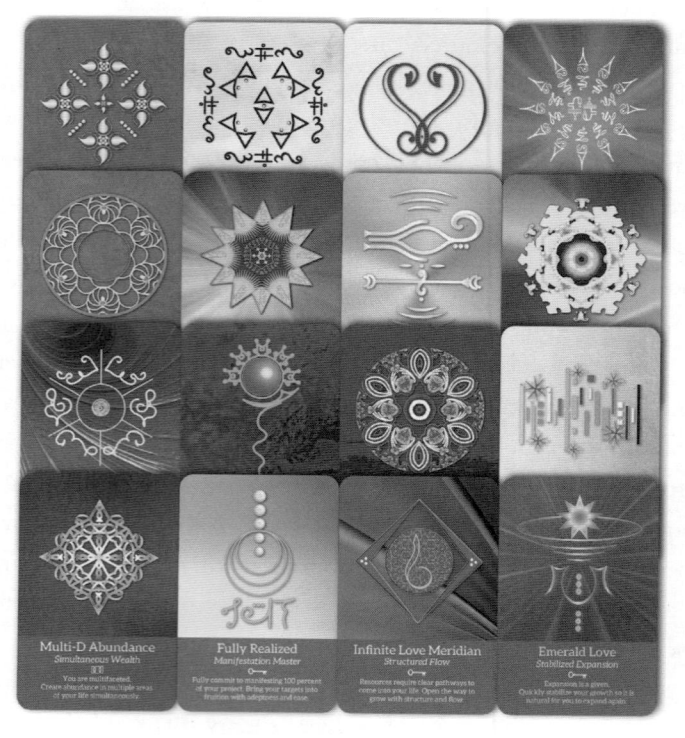

Sixteen-Card Spread

Then from the top of the deck pull out the first card. Place it under the first resource code where it covers the caption box so you only see the glyph of the resource card. Proceed to pull three additional cards so each resource code has one card underneath it. Repeat this process for the next row and continue to place the additional cards to cover the caption box so you are seeing only the glyphs for the first twelve cards. Then on the final row you will see the caption boxes, which represent a summarized message for you about that resource code and your entire Multi-D Abundance spread. It is visually stunning and deeply moving to see the glyphs like a tapestry or patchwork quilt.

YUMMY MONEY SPREADS

Actualize a New Paradigm of Wealth and Create an Extraordinary Partnership with Yummy Money

When you choose to create an energy vortex around money, or when this card comes into your spread, you can experience immediate shifts in your perception, relationship, and internal stance with money. Here is a three-step Yummy Money session to create massive shifts in your inner relationship with money.

Step One: Call Back Energy You May Have Overlaid onto Money

Each time you interact with this code, call back any energy you have placed on money. Reclaim any nuggets of power you have given away to money. Receive back any dreams or aspirations you may have postponed out of the excuse or experience of not enough money. Call back your signature energy and any slower vibrations that you have placed on top of money. When you call back slower vibrations like fear or powerlessness, you reclaim the essence of the energy that is yours in a coherent form, not the illusion or distorted form of energy.

You require all your energy as a creator, from the slowest octaves to the highest octaves, to create what you're here to create. As you commune with the Yummy Money Code, declare that all energy that you may have misplaced, misidentified, projected, separated, divorced from yourself around the subject of money is returned to you with love, grace, and consciousness. Breathe for a few moments as you gaze upon this glyph. Gazing and breathing shifts your internal perception. When you've misplaced energy onto something like money, relationships, energy, or time, and then you reclaim that power and divine qualities, your vibration rises. Your system is amplified, turned up, and turned on.

The first step is that the Yummy Money Code transmits and places your energy on the altar of the heart for you to reclaim again. This is energy that you may have projected onto money. The more energy you have, the more you're coming from a place of wholeness, and the better partner you are to gift, have, and receive money.

Step Two: Offer Up Your Old Money Story and Relationship

Now, as you gaze upon the glyph—which, like all the resource codes is simultaneously a key and hologram glyph in sacred union—you're invited to offer up your old money story. In bringing "yummy" into this code, we've created a sacred union of divine wholeness of money: the Divine Feminine, and Divine Masculine in unity. "Yummy" is a receptive, feminine, juicy, attractive, enjoyable, pleasurable, divine quality and experience. And "money" is often thought of as masculine energy, at least when it becomes physicalized. Of course, money is money in wholeness. Having "yummy" and "money" together creates a structured flow. It creates a sacred union of wholeness.

Place your old story around money as an offering for future generations to learn from on the altar of the infinite source of money, which is Source. These would be all disappointments, frustrations, and fears, and also what you perceive as the good aspects of your old money story. Regardless, put your old story on the altar so you can create an extraordinary partnership with money. This happens quickly and in alignment with your free will and conscious choice. It occurs in a very aligned and rapid way. Are you willing to have a brand-new relationship with money?

In step one, you have reclaimed your energy and power. In step two, you place on the altar the source of all money, your outdated relationship with money, and any old-paradigm money stories pertaining to lack or scarcity.

Step Three: Create a Loving Partnership with Yummy Money

Now you're open to a new partnership with the Yummy Money being. As you create an energetic container for your partnership with money contemplate what the foundation of that partnership might be. What qualities matter to you in your relationship with money? Perhaps it's joy, magic, generosity, surplus, or prosperity. Maybe for you, money is about being so well nourished that your big mission has all the resources it requires.

What would you place on the altar of your inner relationship with Yummy Money? Are you open to money doing things for you? Are you ready to have money champion your creations? Are you willing for money to be a vehicle for impeccable self-care? Step one, reclaim your energy. Step two, offer up your old stories. Step three, declare your new feeling tone in your partnership with money.

For example, when Yummy Money comes into your financial containers it is imbued with a win, win, win for all involved. Everything you touch turns to gold and is expanded. Money pools around you and desires to hang out with you. You have clarity about when to circulate and receive money and when to grow it.

When you upgrade your internal relationship with money you shift outdated perceptions such as, "I don't have enough. I can't depend on money. Whatever comes in goes out. I have past disappointments of wanting money and it didn't show up." Instead, you create a clean slate. And not only that, your relationship with money is one of the best relationships you have based on mutual honoring and bringing out the best in one another. You are the biggest cheerleaders for each other. When you and Yummy Money partner together, your mission thrives, and you cocreate tremendous good in the world.

Create Financial Abundance

Now that you've shifted your internal communion with money let's move into creating money in the outer planes. Be very specific about what you're choosing to have, create, and actualize when it comes to money. This includes both the internal way you relate to money, like yumminess, and the external containers for financial abundance, like the money in your bank. Maybe you're dedicating your card spread to up your annual income, build your net worth, or have a business with a certain profit level.

Be clear about what you're choosing to have in your external money containers. It may be net worth, income, paying off debt, investments, real estate, cash, gold, or silver. These are all forms of expression of Yummy Money. Be clear about the external abundance you're choosing to create and why you desire it, so that when Yummy Money comes into your energy vortexes, it has a direction and a home.

These four resource codes are interconnected. Perhaps your Yummy Money reason for having more passive income is that you'll have more time to spend your way, which falls under the banner of Sublime Time. Perhaps the Yummy Money is related to hiring someone to help you with your business or your kids, which is a Divine Relationship resource code. You may notice Yummy Money and Radiant Energy increasing simultaneously. The fear of not having enough, lack, and doubt that may have been draining your Radiant Energy may become radiant again. These resources are interconnected. Build a direct relationship with the money being. Be clear, and direct the energy of money to receive, gift, and have financial wealth on the physical plane.

SUBLIME TIME SPREADS
Unlock Your Sublime Time Treasure Chest

Use this spread when you have an intention to manifest a new dimension of time, like taking back one day a week to spend your way—or speeding up the time it takes to complete a project, like writing a book in half the time. When you've got a lot on your plate, collapse time, jump timelines, and stretch and bend time by pulling cards for Sublime Time. Declare "I have more than enough time, everything gets done, and it all doesn't have to be done by me." Intend that each moment is sublime and nourishing rather than depleting. Experience a cornucopia of synchronicities and enjoy your tasks as they are magically completed.

Create an altar to calibrate your day to the optimal outcomes for your projects and manifestations. Replace outdated patterns—of overworking, micromanaging, or trying to control everything—with Heart-Sentience and a sense of ease. As you create from love you leverage the universe's divine order.

Let's say you have twenty things on your to-do list, and maybe five of those involve calling someone to follow up on something. Create a Sublime Time vortex, and perhaps those individuals call you, or other items on your list get done in less time than you had blocked out and then you have the space to make the calls. Rather than doing eight thousand, eighty, or eight action steps to create an outcome, an external manifestation, or actualization, Sublime Time circumvents the actions that aren't necessary.

Create a Sublime Time altar when you notice your energy waning or you're feeling zapped. Or create it at times when you haven't had or chosen to take as much time as you'd like to nourish yourself with hobbies, friends, or exercise. Take five minutes to lie down and do a Sublime Time altar spread. Maybe you take great pleasure in spending time with a friend you haven't seen in a while. During that five minutes, imagine you're spending time together in the higher planes—in alignment with that person's free will and conscious choice. If you love rock climbing and you haven't been rock climbing, for that five minutes of Sublime Time, bilocate to rock climb and receive the nourishment from it on the multidimensional and Earth plane.

Use Sublime Time spreads to collapse or bend time and jump onto your highest timeline. Create energy vortexes to access off-planet lifetimes, gifts, and talents. Leverage time by cocreating with others so that more things get done without you being the one who does them, receiving more without doing more. Those are beautiful Sublime Time altars that allow other possibilities to bubble up within you.

DIVINE RELATIONSHIPS SPREADS
Call In or Upgrade Relationships

Personal Relationship Spreads

Relationships are one of the most significant resources you have. You can do a manifestation spread to meet somebody new or up-level your current relationships. Maybe a long-term relationship has stopped growing. Or perhaps there is conflict in a relationship, family, or group of individuals. Create an altar to upgrade these relationships, to open the flow of love within them so that they become extraordinary again.

Perhaps you desire to call in new relationships—deeper friendships, community, a significant other, or a four-legged friend. Create an energy vortex with this purpose in mind. Look at the cards you've drawn several times a day and bring up the feelings of connection, love, fun, or other qualities you desire in the relationship. Or create a trio of abundance spread and leave it on your nightstand while you sleep in order to call in your next-level partnerships.

You can go even deeper by homing in on a particular aspect of the relationship, like communication or clarity. You can create a Divine Relationships energy vortex for your health, body, and energy. Dedicate a spread to your relationship with the masculine or men you have relationships with like your brother, father, or spouse. Bring healing to your relationship with the feminine by creating an altar with the women you have in your life like your sister, mother, or significant other. You can also call upon the Divine Relationships code and consecrate an energy vortex to an institution like marriage. Let's say your parents are divorced and you're engaged. Your knowledge that 50 percent of marriages end in divorce clouds your idea of marriage.

Create an altar to cultivate a Divine Relationship with the institution of marriage.

Don't stop there. Instead, create energy vortexes for your relationship with food, money, or your home. Do spreads for your relationships with yourself, your guides, pets, and especially your relationship with your manifestation projects. There are infinite possibilities. Tap into your inner knowing and have fun with these spreads.

When the Divine Relationships Code steps forward, connect to the power of the "we"—the energetic aspect of the relationship. In any relationship, there is you, and someone or something else, ideally as two whole autonomous beings. The relationship is a third thing between the two of you. Honor the "we." Send love and appreciation and nourishment to the "we" of the relationship being. The relationship is the third point of attraction for your creations to find you.

Nourish and be present to your relationship with your project, the "we" between you, and the love being that is your manifestation. Notice your operating system with this project you're manifesting. Have you been overgiving, overdoing things, or micromanaging? Have you been playing small, hiding out, holding back, or being invisible? Have you been deferring your power to others? No matter what you've been doing, you can shift this now to bring spring green newness, fresh energy, and new beginnings back into your projects and relationships.

All expressions of relationships are extensions of Source energy. They may be coherent expressions of Source energy or distorted expressions overlaid onto Source energy. When this card comes into your spreads there is a recalibration to coherence. Like all the Magdalene Codes, this resource code is power packed with love. Any disempowering behavior you may have been indulging in your relationships, is, at its base, due to an absence of love.

Let this Divine Relationships Code unlock overflowing love within you and your manifestations. Know that even though it may be a big step to open to Divine Relationships, it's a necessary one to actualize 100 percent of your manifestations and to become Fully Realized in this lifetime. Ask this code to support you and be willing to be willing to have the abundance of Divine Partnerships, and watch your creations flourish!

Professional Relationship Spreads

Divine Relationships is a go-to spread when you're looking to enhance your current relationships and call in new individuals to help leverage your time and fully achieve your mission. If you're a transformational entrepreneur and hiring, pull out your card deck and create a Divine Relationships altar. Dedicate the energy vortex to call in your perfectly matched team member and upgrade your current partnerships with team members, collaborators, or vendors.

If you have a service and you're calling in soul-aligned clients, create a spread to fill your programs using the airwaves of energy and multidimensional communication. This allows your energy vortex and the love body of your program to broadcast a clear signal to those who are a vibrational match for you. Telepathic communication amplifies the aligned action you are taking.

Creating energy vortexes that involve others is always in alignment with the free will and conscious choice of those involved to choose to partner with you and you with them—or not. All manifestations are in divine order and in adherence to the universal principles of the highest and best good of all.

RADIANT ENERGY SPREADS
Regenerate, Rejuvenate, and Renew

Radiant Energy spreads help you replenish, rejuvenate, and regenerate your system and shift out of fatigue and burnout. Create a card spread to assist you in feeling ten years younger. Shift out of the illusion lie that as you age your body and energy have to deteriorate.

Perhaps a lack of Radiant Energy is your impetus for the creation spread. Remember with all your manifesting that even if the desire for more seems to stem from lack consciousness—

you're tired so you want energy, or you're lonely so you want relationships—the lack energy that brought you to the spread is not the energy you sprinkle into your creation vortex. You're not creating from a vibration of lack. You're starting from a place of being resourced. That's why we call these "resource codes"; you are re-Sourced.

You can dedicate your Radiant Energy spreads to different expressions of your energy. Maybe at the end of your workday, you're zapped. Create a Radiant Energy spread to be rejuvenated and nourished while you're at work, and have more energy at the end of the day than when you began. Maybe as a parent you've been not sleeping well. Cultivate a Radiant Energy vortex for deeply nourishing sleep for you and your family, in alignment with their free will.

We're speaking about your 3D reality, but you and the resource codes are multidimensional. What you choose to manifest with the assistance of the Magdalene Codes is based on multiple dimensions of your focus, including your choice, decision, the energy of surplus, the new paradigm, and multidimensionality.

A possible origin of having a lack of energy is that you may be primarily experiencing yourself and your life through slower vibrational thoughts, feelings, and sensations—doubt, fear, survival consciousness—rather than being fully tapped into your multidimensionality beyond the third dimensional identity of body, mind, emotion. You are more than these three dimensions. You are a divine being, multidimensional with abundant eternal Radiant Energy. We know that the process of experiencing yourself from your human perspective to fully embodying your divine self is an evolution in consciousness and physical radiance. Our flagstaff programs, Divine Light Activation and the Magdalene Codes program, assist with this multidimensional living. The Magdalene Codes program is an opportunity to work more deeply with these codes (see the What's Next section for more information).

Create a Radiant Energy altar to tap into the resource of nonphysical energy—your soul, higher self, light being self, and love being self that fuels you and your love body. Dedicate a Radiant Energy spread to your relationship with your higher self. You could dedicate a Radiant Energy spread as well to one of the dimensions of your 3D identity, like your emotions, your body, or your thoughts, which play a massive role in how energetic you feel or don't feel.

Create an energy vortex for having Radiant Energy thoughts. Notice what you're saying to yourself that depletes your energy. How often do you think things like *I'm tired* or find yourself worrying about not having enough energy to get through the day? Do a spread to amplify appreciative thoughts that grow your energy and anchor, imbue, and seal in this way of being as a given. This way you're tapped into the infinite supply of Radiant Energy, regenerating and rejuvenating in all now-moments.

Create new neuropathways around feeling energized with a "leap while you sleep" trio of abundance spread that you put next to you while sleeping. When you awaken, rather than being sluggish, you're refreshed, renewed, and ready to embrace the day with pep in your step. A lot of what shifts this is what you say to yourself. Spend a few minutes in appreciation and gratitude before getting up.

Most likely it's not only slower vibrational thoughts that drain you, it's a combo platter of your emotions and body sensations. Maybe there has been worry, fear, anger, depression, or doubt that created symptoms like insomnia or pain in your body. You can do a spread to be passionate and have a zest for life, to be in a state of joy and appreciation for your life exactly as it is.

Creating manifestation spreads for your internal states is a revolutionary aspect of the Magdalene Codes. We are not only inviting you to focus your manifestation on creating on the external plane. Those are absolutely a part of the picture; however, they're not the entire picture, for you are also meant to enjoy the journey along the way. You can do a card spread to cultivate a new emotional set point or feeling tone—a dominant positive feeling throughout the day. Your elevated mood propagates uplifting thoughts and supports your body to be an instrument of higher consciousness rather than running on a cocktail of stress hormones.

You can do a manifestation spread for installing new beliefs, new emotional set points, or new body experiences. For example: that your digestive system is humming and thrumming. It may be that you do a Radiant Energy spread for body alignment or to be deeply nourished and fueled. Sleep, exercise, food, and water nourish your body. However, your body may be asking for Star Love or Emerald Love.

Use the Radiant Energy spreads to summon resources that regenerate your system and fuel your soul or your multidimensional self. Open up to even greater radiance. Rest, renew, and rejuvenate with the support of Radiant Energy.

Conclusion
Deepening Your Magdalene Manifestation Practice

Now that you're tapped into the higher purpose of a manifestation practice to not only include the joy of creating in the material plane and re-Sourcing your mission in this lifetime but also to be a rapid path to union with Source, things get a lot more interesting. Applying spiritual truths on Earth by creating abundance is a way you embody and live higher states of consciousness. As well it's a path of becoming your highest self through love.

Remember to call upon us in your manifestation practice, for we are part of your council cheering you on from the higher dimensions. Your life is overflowing with synchronicities, magic, and optimal experiences that guide you all along the way. Steeping in the Magdalene Codes cards is a process of reclaiming dominion of your multidimensionality and a return to wholeness. It is our joy and delight to be participating in the larger movement in consciousness into love. We are extending our love, appreciation, and acknowledgment to you for your contribution to the evolution in consciousness. It takes all of us and is a joy to do together.

We'll see you in the codes and be with you during your manifestation spreads and energy vortexes as your manifestations go from the process of morphing from being Love Conceptions into Fully Realized Magdalene Love Beings. Create for the pure joy of it! You are a creator love being.

> ALL IS LIGHT AND LOVE AND WE ARE ALL,
> THE MAGDALENE MIDWIVES

P.S. If you'd like to go deeper with the codes be sure to check out our What's Next section to access additional tools and explore how we can continue to partner together.

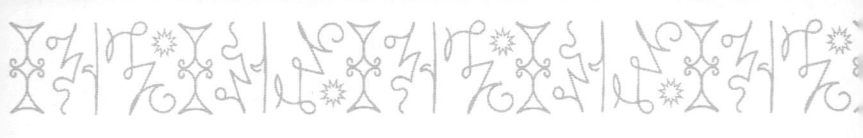

What's Next
Explore Additional Ways to Work with the Magdalenes

This is the Magdalenes, Thoth, and the Council of Light moving into the forefront of this divine transmission. We are delighted to place the invitation to continue to partner with us on the altar for you to pick up if it is aligned for you. Do you sense we may have a divine appointment to connect further? Are you vibrationally recognizing that what you have been asking for and what we are sharing is a match? If so, please enjoy the following gifts and explore our signature programs. We look forward to connecting further.

THE MAGDALENES, THOTH, AND
THE COUNCIL OF LIGHT

Additional Tools for Your Journey

Meet the Magdalenes Channeled Guided Meditation
Communicating with light beings isn't as hard as you think. You have a unique Magdalene Council of love beings, a manifestation team in light, who are delighted to support you as you create abundance through love. This channeled audio assists

you in forging and deepening an authentic partnership with the Magdalenes and your higher self-guidance as you work with this deck. To access this guided meditation, visit www.DanielleHoffman.com/Magdalene.

Magdalene Codes Affirmations Reference Sheet

You may find having an overview of the names of the codes and their associated glyphs and affirmations all in one place incredibly useful to see the big picture of the entire manifestation system and accelerate your results.

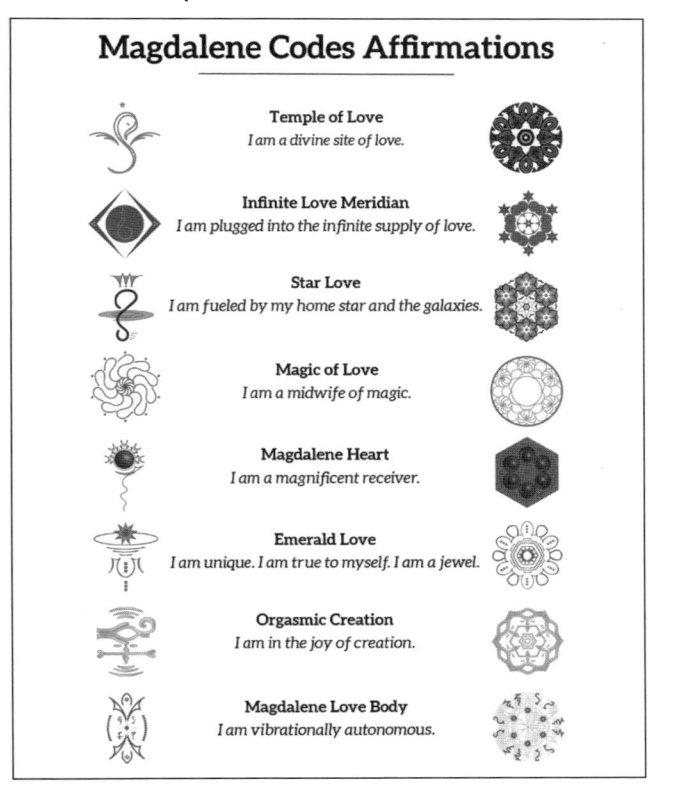

Magdalene Codes Affirmations

Temple of Love
I am a divine site of love.

Infinite Love Meridian
I am plugged into the infinite supply of love.

Star Love
I am fueled by my home star and the galaxies.

Magic of Love
I am a midwife of magic.

Magdalene Heart
I am a magnificent receiver.

Emerald Love
I am unique. I am true to myself. I am a jewel.

Orgasmic Creation
I am in the joy of creation.

Magdalene Love Body
I am vibrationally autonomous.

If you'd enjoy having this affirmation sheet for quick reference, you can download it at www.DanielleHoffman.com/Magdalene.

Yummy Money Workshop

This workshop explores the energetic secrets on how to be wildly magnetic to money, how to grow spiritually with money, and what your body and nervous system require so that money stays and builds in your life. In this online channeled workshop, the Magdalenes and I reveal the exact energetic adjustments I downloaded from the guides, which took me from being burned out at six-figures to radiant at seven-figures. In the spirit of abundance, with the purchase of this guidebook you receive access to a complimentary Yummy Money workshop at www.DanielleHoffman.com/Magdalene.

Embody Your Divine Self: Explore Our Core Programs

In our abundant array of core programs and masterclasses, we help new practitioners and seasoned spiritual coaches and healers manifest abundance, reconnect with Source, and fulfill their divine assignment in this incarnation. We offer direct activation work with Danielle and the Magdalenes as well as accelerated programs hand-delivered from the Ascended Masters to activate and embody your Divine self, mission, and leadership.

Magdalene Codes Expanded Curriculum

If you'd like to dive deeper into the Magdalene Codes work you've begun with this deck, you can get started with the

Magdalene Masterclass and/or take the full program to become a fully activated Magdalene Love Being:

- Magdalene Birthright of Love Masterclass: Crack the 5D Time Code to Take Back Your Life (Fridays Off, Unplugged Vacations, Space to Create)
- Magdalene Codes of Love: Expand your capacity to receive more and create quantum leaps in your money, time, relationships, and energy without overworking or experiencing a body crash

In this potent container of the full Magdalene Codes program you will work directly with the Magdalenes and Danielle to cultivate your ability to receive more and expand again. You will create your unique Multi-D Abundance temple, including the four resources of Yummy Money (add 2k, 20k, or 200k to your money containers), Sublime Time (take back one day a week to spend your way—three-day weekends with your family, yoga on the beach, finally writing that book, or getting the certification you're passionate about), Divine Relationships (aligned clients, team, community, connected to Source every day), and Radiant Energy (highly magnetic, feel ten years younger, bountiful energy to get it all done). By the end of our time together, you will have activated all the Magdalene Codes in your system—a complete initiation as a Magdalene Love Being.

Spiritual Mentorship Programs
- Divine Light Activation: Lead Your Highest Mission as an Embodied Divine Being

- Ascended Master Academy: Create Your Legacy-Work (Unique Modality, Book, Program, Business) with Source
- Sahu—Be Your Fully Realized Self: A Year of Enlightenment with the Ascended Masters

To find out more about these offerings, including advanced spiritual mentorship and live events, go to www.DanielleHoffman.com.

About the Author and the Artist

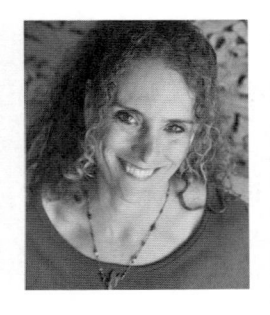

Author Danielle Rama Hoffman

Danielle Rama Hoffman is a bestselling author, international channel, and legacy-work coach to thousands around the world. She is the cocreator (with her guides) of the Magdalene Codes of Love, Divine Light Activation, the Ascended Master Academy, and the Sahu Embodiment Program, where her specialty is leading seasoned and emerging coaches, healers, mentors, and spiritual teachers to embody their Divine self and create their UNIQUE legacy body of work (book, program, business) with Source.

Since 1994 Danielle has been leading the evolution in consciousness and is an advocate for lightworkers sharing their highest mission prosperously without overworking or fear of visibility getting in the way. Her clients are high performing, dialed-in spiritual beings who are committed to expanding consciousness and making a difference on the planet and span from experts in their field (university teachers, doctors, corporate executives), spiritual growth adepts (retired, or stay at home moms), and transformational entrepreneurs (healers, coaches, practitioners) starting or growing their business.

To find out about current ways to continue to work more deeply with Danielle, Thoth, the Ascended Masters, and the Magdalenes go to DanielleHoffman.com. To read more books from Danielle, including the light trilogy (*The Council of Light, The Tablets of Light,* and *The Temples of Light*) go to www.innertraditions.com/author/danielle-rama-hoffman.

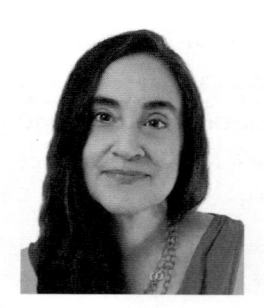

Artist Christine Lucas

The symbols on these cards were created by artist and intuitive Christine Lucas, who translated the energies of the Codes of Love into shape, geometry, and color. Christine has partnered deeply with Thoth and Divine Transmissions over the years and is part of the Ascended Masters Lineage of Thoth. She scribed these beautiful symbols in multidimensional partnership with Thoth, the Magdalenes, the Codes of Love, and Danielle. You can learn more about her work at www.ChristineLucasArt.com.